Best Tips For Women Dayhikers:

Everything You Need To Know To Hit The Trail

Diane Spicer

Hiking For Her

Table of Contents

Author

Diane Spicer has been hiking a long, long time.

Don't believe it?

Subtract 1970 from the current year, and there you have it.

She fell in love with soggy hiking trails on Isle Royale National Park in Lake Superior, and in the Porcupine Mountains in the western half of Michigan's Upper Peninsula.

From there, she branched out to drier, higher trails in the western United States, Canada, and Greenland.

To say she's a passionate hiker is a huge understatement.

Hiking defines her, consumes her, drives her to learn more and more about how to get the most out of trail time.

Add to this hiking passion some advanced degrees in education and human biology, and you've got a highly experienced teacher for the art and science of hiking in a female human body.

Preface

Welcome to **Best Hiking Tips For Women Dayhikers!**

It's me, Diane Spicer from Hiking For Her, here to welcome you and to let you know what's in store for you in these pages.

The hiking tips in this book can be blamed on my addiction to hiking.

My obsession with hiking began innocently enough, with an invitation to join a Girl Scout backpacking trip to Isle Royale National Park in Lake Superior. Let's leave the date a bit vague, but call it 1970-ish.

Give a girl a backpack, and she's gonna want boots. Give her sturdy boots, and she's gonna want a compass.

You get the idea!

Five decades later, I'm still hiking, but now I'm writing down my best hiking tips for hikers. What a rewarding way to reach out to my virtual hiking partners, via the Hiking For Her website (please visit www.hiking-for-her.com).

Every email I receive leads me down another path, literally or figuratively, and more pages of hiking tips get written as a result.

But over the years, these hiking tips have really piled up (over 350 pages and growing). It's getting to be a challenge to find exactly what you need in the maze of interconnected hiking tips.

The search box at the bottom of each page on the website helps you navigate.

So does selecting "site map" on the navigation bar on the left hand side of each web page.

But I'm guessing that you want something a little faster when you have questions about day hiking.

That's what this book is designed to give you: Ten chapters of Hiking For Her's best tips for day hikers, pulled together in one spot and organized for your convenience.

A quick peek at the Table of Contents shows you what's in store for you: solid information on hiking gear and techniques to use before, during and after a dayhike.

These tips have been gathered from Hiking For Her's extensive website pages, and then edited, enhanced and clarified to streamline your reading experience.

In the e-book edition, in each chapter you will find several types of links to additional information.

-Some links take you to pages on the HFH website, giving you further details and background information that would make this book too long.

Don't click the link unless you want to divert off the trail! But remember, diversions can be fun.

-Some of the links will take you to a website, pdf download, map or other free resource that will make your trail time safer and more enjoyable.

-A third set of links will be found at the end of every chapter, tantalizing you with more resources, recommendations and additional information that didn't quite fit in the streamlined chapter.

But in this hard copy version, you will find this information at the end of each chapter. It's organized by key words so you can visit the Hiking For Her website and search for each topic.

Before we get started with hiking tips, let's define a dayhiker so we're both on the same page (which we should be, after all this IS a book).

A dayhiker:

-wakes up at home or at a campsite;

-eats breakfast and journeys to a trailhead (maybe simultaneously);

-hikes at least a few hours but could stay on the trail as long as there's daylight;

-prefers good weather and maintained trails with adequate signage;

-has a definite turn around spot (or time) in mind;

-carries a light weight day pack with food, water and other essentials;

-leaves the trail before dark, with no intention of camping overnight.

So what kind of dayhiker would need the best hiking tips offered in this book?

Well, if you're just starting out as a dayhiker, you will save yourself a ton of time and money by reading and applying these hiking tips. Use a "learn as you go" approach, with this book as your mentor.

Been day hiking for a while but have a few gear, navigation, or food issues that you'd like to solve or improve? Use this book as a rich resource to fine tune your approach to the trail.

Can you see that I really mean it when I say that *HFH gives you hiking advice you can trust*? I've gathered together a treasure trove of hiking tips and resources for your enjoyment.

Comments, feed back, suggestions, photos of your hikes, a note to say hi – those are also welcome and appreciated via the CONTACT link on the website.

Thanks for the chance to walk with you down the trail, if only for a little virtual while.

May all of your trails bring you good things.

-Diane Spicer

Hiking For Her

P.S. The cover photo was taken on a day hike in the Canadian Rockies by David Midkiff, my husband and intrepid trail buddy.

The HFH website has many more of his photos of enticing hiking destinations, alpine flowers, and lots more for you to enjoy!

Before Your Day Hike

Putting yourself "out there" on a hiking trail is an expression of your adventurous spirit.

But along with that exhilarating sense of adventure, you need to control the essential factors that make you a dayhiker: footwear, backpack, hiking clothes, trail food, planning your destination and more.

Having firm control over these variables puts you in a position of strength to deal with unpredictable events like nasty weather, animal encounters, and misadventures in map reading.

It also makes your day hike much more enjoyable.

In this section, you'll learn all of the details in these essential factors for a successful day hike, one chapter at a time. There's no need to read these chapters in order, but I do recommend that you read them all before you hit the trail.

Chapter 1: Day Hike Gear

Chapter 2: Hiking Ten Essentials

Chapter 3: Trail Nutrition

Chapter 4: Hydration

Chapter 5: Destination and Itinerary

Don't forget to dip into the Resources at the end of each chapter.

Ready to dive in?

Great!

Here we go!

Chapter 1: Day Hike Gear

The right gear keeps you happy and safe on a trail, but it doesn't have to be the most expensive or most elaborate hiking gear on the market.

The most important criteria? It must *fit you well* and *enhance your trail time* (rather than hold you back).

So how will you find this "just right" gear? Read this chapter!

You'll find the answers to these important dayhiking considerations:

Footwear: Boots or shoes?

Socks: One pair or two?

Pack: How big do I need?

Hiking clothing: Why build a layering system of breathable wicking fabrics?

Sports bra and underwear: What to look for beyond color and fit?

Trekking poles: When and how to use them?

Let's start off on the right foot, shall we? (Or left foot, your choice.)

FOOTWEAR

The first thing you probably thought about when you began to get interested in day hiking was what to put on your feet.

And that's ***exactly the place to start*** when you're building your gear list, because the comfort of your feet will make or break your hike.

Blisters, pinched toes, foot cramps – who needs them? Not happy hikers!

Today's advanced technology puts many choices of trail footwear literally at your feet: lightweight breathable hiking boots, heavy soled rugged leather hiking boots, low cut hiking shoes, as well as minimalist trail running shoes.

Maybe too many choices! So let's keep it simple: What's on your feet depends on the type of trail you've picked out for your day hike.

We'll assume that you're not carrying much weight, and that you're dedicated to the idea of gracefully meeting whatever the trail throws at you: rocks, roots, mud, tree branches, uneven footing, steep inclines, and more.

To fully understand trail footwear, you'll need some terms: minimalist, low profile, traditional, and maximum.

You'll also need a few guidelines to make choosing your first pair of boots or trail shoes as easy and painless as possible.

Let's wade through these terms and guidelines so you understand your options for footwear.

-**Lightweight hiking boots** (traditional) are best for varied trail conditions, thanks to their sturdy yet lightweight upper construction.

You can select thin or thick soles, depending on what you've got planned.

Wear these on hikes where you rely on a grooved sole for traction, and water resistance against modest amounts of mud, roots, puddles or shallow stream crossings.

These boots provide a decent amount of ankle and arch support, important if you aren't used to uneven terrain.

And nothing makes you feel like a "real" hiker than your first pair of hiking boots!

-**Heavy soled leather hiking boots** (maximum) will protect your feet from rocky terrain.

Their heavy Vibram (rubber) soles give you a rock solid grip on sloped, sandy or pebbled surfaces, and keep your feet dry if you have to cross shallow rushing streams or wade through boggy areas.

You will definitely feel these boots on your feet!

Sturdy boots like these also give maximum support and stability under heavy loads, but this probably doesn't apply to you as a day hiker unless you plan to lug slabs of granite off the mountain (ha!).

-**Hiking shoes** (low profile) are designed with a lower cut and featherweight mesh uppers, but don't have rugged soles.

Choose these for only the best trail conditions: dry, flat trail hiking with a lightweight pack, for example.

Expect to replace them more frequently than boots, because they aren't designed to stand up to roots, rocks or lots of moisture.

If you hike frequently, you'll find yourself traveling over rougher terrain and will notice the tread diminish rather quickly.

You might also begin wishing for more support and protection than shoes can provide to you.

-**Trail running shoes** (low profile) tell you exactly when to use them. However, if you're going to do trail running as well as dayhiking, you might not need two sets of footwear.

Test one pair of trail running shoes under both conditions and see if you are satisfied with their support, traction and comfort. Only your feet will know for sure.

-**Trail sandals** (minimalist) are not recommended by Hiking For Her for some very compelling reasons, including the safety of your feet and the annoyance of gritty pokey things between your toes.

But they do have their uses! If you're going to do a lot of stream crossings, carry a lightweight, fast drying pair of sandals strapped to the outside of your pack and don them when needed.

But please don't risk your feet on the trail in open toed, non supportive sandals. You don't want to lose any skin to the trail.

You can head over to the RESOURCES section at the end of Chapter One to view examples of each of these categories of footwear.

As you can see, the right hiking footwear is going to change with your evolving day hiking needs. But here's a good summary statement:

The more casual the trail and the lighter the pack, the lighter the footwear required.

The caveat: Lightweight footwear, while less expensive, will need to be replaced more frequently.

Time To Shop!

Now that you've decided which category of trail footwear you need, you're probably eager to go shopping.

Tip: It's best to go to a "bricks and mortar" store the first time you buy hiking footwear.

Why? You want to try out different brands. And you definitely want to open each box and take a close look at potential trail wear with these questions in mind:

1. How easy is it to get these on and off? (**laces/lacing system**)

2. What kind of grip will they have on the trail? (**soles**)

3. Can they accommodate my particular arch, width of foot, and any foot issues I have? (**toe box, arch support and cushioning**)

4. How wet will my feet get if I really push these? (**water repellent - vs- water proof**)

The subtext of these questions: *How comfortable will they be?*

The answer revolves around the amount of trail wear required for your feet to mold your footwear choices to your distinctive footprint. Think of this as "break in time". It can be measured in hours for lightweight footwear, or weeks to months for stiff leather boots.

This time frame is important if you are going to be doing a lot of dayhiking within a short period of time, but haven't given yourself a lot of break in time.

If you need right-out-of-the-box comfort, try on trail shoes with a low profile and plenty of flexibility.

Lightweight boots will offer more support than shoes and should be comfy right out of the box, if they are well fitted. They outshine heavier boots in terms of reducing leg fatigue, but are deficient in protecting your feet and ankles from trail hazards such as spiny plants, jagged rocks, and uneven surfaces.

If you have time to acclimate to boots and "break them in", leather boots will give you maximum support and protection on the trail. Just realize that it will take a few hikes to adjust to their stiffness and to achieve an acceptable level of comfort as they mold to the contours of your feet.

An important note about "weak" ankles: If you're prone to ankle injuries, including any tendency to roll or strain or sprain or twist them, you probably need more support in your trail footwear. Opt for boots over shoes, and lace them up correctly (see Chapter 1 Resources) to provide adequate ankle support.

Side note: The more you hike, the stronger your legs will become. This can cut down on your tendency toward "weak" ankles. And in turn, you can try lighter, less supportive footwear.

If you're looking to invest in footwear that will last for multiple seasons, avoid shoes and look at boots. The amount of materials, combined with the quality and durability of components, will disappoint you in hiking shoes if you plan to wrack up lots of mileage.

On the other hand, if you don't mind replacing trail shoes more frequently, you'll always have the latest lightweight technology and styling to keep your feet comfortable.

And as long as you don't carry a lot of weight in your pack, you can trade support and traction for that high level of immediate comfort – right out of the box.

How To Size Up A Pair Of Boots

Let's take a quick tour through a pair of hiking boots, pointing out the essential features to pay attention to when you open up the box and try them on.

1. **SOLES:**

If you plan to use these boots for flat trail hiking in dry weather, you don't need to be concerned about "grippy" soles. But if your hikes will take you to uneven and steep terrain in wet conditions, you will find yourself depending upon their gripping ability in a big way.

To be truthful, every hiker faces these types of conditions sooner or later. So "grippy" soles are important to all of us.

Grip is all about the contours on the bottom of the boot, so be sure to turn over the boot and check out the depth of tread on the sole.

If you're a newbie dayhiker, shallow smooth soles will give you adequate traction for beginning level trails.

But if you plan to become a more aggressive day hiker, or will make unplanned detours off the trail due to blow downs or animal activity, you'll need the tread to match your pursuits. For these reasons, seek out the boots with deepest tread for your anticipated needs.

You also want *non-uniform distribution* of the tread. This ensures that trail debris doesn't have a chance to build up and rob you of traction and sensitivity to the trail conditions. Who likes to go skidding across pea sized gravel on a slope, or slide across wet talus piles?

Tip: Please believe me when I say that tread is important for all but the most flat well behaved trails. So every season, check the tread just as you'd check the tread on your car tires.

For the best tread available, look for rubber soles made out of Vibram; they are durable and notoriously "sticky". There are other rubber blends with different names which also deliver gripalong with durability.

Bottom line for soles: look for durability, but know that the more rugged soles will push the cost of the boot upward.

Cost -vs- durability, that's the puzzle you need to solve for yourself.

2. FABRICS/MATERIALS:

Will these bootsstand up to what you are going to throw at them? You can answer yes if they are water repellent or water proof, durable, breathable, and well made by reputable manufacturers.

Read the information supplied with the boots, scanning for trade names such as Gore-tex (known for water resistance and breathability), Cordura, linings such as Cambrelle, and Thinsulate.

Here's one more reason why it pays to goto a store with trained sales people. They can answer your questions, show you literature from the manufacturer, and hopefully share their own experiences with selecting best hiking boots for all sorts of feet.

If they can't do that, or have an unfriendly attitude, take your business elsewhere. I don't know about you, but I wouldn't buy a car from someone who doesn't drive. Why buy hiking boots from someone who doesn't hike?

The flip side, of course, is keeping these stores in the business of supplying you with great hiking gear. Buy directly from gear stores that treat you right, because if you don't, they will close their doors and your hiking gear will have to come from places you have no relationship with. That's a lose-lose proposition in the long run.

3. INSERTS:

Look for removable inserts - a great plus when you need to dry out your boots after crossing a soggy meadow.

These inserts will conform to the contours of your feet after a few times out on the trail (the good news), and will need to be replaced every so often in order to maintain a good fit (the bad news).

Another use of the word "insert" may refer to an optional piece of molded material inserted into a boot for a more customized fit. The boot store will likely carry these inserts (at additional cost) to customize your boots, and can guide you as to what you need based on your foot structure.

If you don't like the idea of spending more money to get a great fit, skip that particular boot brand.

Or you can try Dr. Scholl's or some other inserts from the nearest drugstore. These inserts are less expensive, can be cut to fit, and are easy to remove and replace. However, they wear out quickly.

Again, cost -vs- durability.

4. LACES & GROMMETS:

Be sure you can easily replace your boot laces once you remove a broken/frayed lace.

What are the chances of the laces wearing out before the soles? Hard to tell, but in my experience, the laces are fairly long lived and will fray only if the grommets are sharp edged or you're hiking in rocky terrain.

The more exposure to extreme temperatures and ultraviolet radiation they endure, the shorter their lifespan.

Always carry a spare set of laces in your pack if you're doing long, hard day hikes. They can be used for many emergency repairs even if you never need them for your boots. And on the day you need them for your boots, you'll be glad you carry them.

Exception: Some trail footwear has a lacing system, with a closed loop of laces that are hard to replace but can stand up to a lot of abuse. And that makes having to replace these laces rather unlikely.

Tips For Boot Buying

Now for some general tips for buying *the* best hiking boots for your hard working feet.

*Shop at the end of a long active day, when your feet are at their maximum dimensions.

*Width and length vary a LOT by manufacturer. Your "normal" shoe size won't automatically be the right fit, because you'll be wearing thicker hiking socks (to be discussed shortly).

Don't be embarrassed (or in denial) if you need a size (or 2) larger - it's only a number! You want high performing feet, right?

Again, here's where it pays to go to a reputable boot dealer with knowledgeable staff who will take the time to work with you on a good fit. They know all the tricks for determining if a boot fits.

*Bring the socks you'll be wearing on the trail, and orthotics (prescribed by a podiatrist) if you require them.

*Walk around for *at least 15 minutes* in the boots, trying to simulate uphill and downhill hiking. Get on your tippy toes, do some heel walking, practice sideways stepping, and throw in a few ankle twists.

Better yet, actually walk on stairs, if the sales folks are amenable.

Some stores (REI gear coop, for instance) have simulated trail terrain for testing. You can even trot over to the backpack department, borrow a loaded backpack, and walk around the store in the prospective boots for awhile.

*Be sure you can return/exchange the boots within a reasonable period of time if they don't work out.

*Consider renting boots from the store if you are a complete newcomer to hiking boots. This gives you a chance to try out various brands before making an expensive commitment. If the thought of wearing pre-worn sweaty boots makes you squirm, realize that you'll be wearing 2 pairs of socks!

*Once you locate the magic combination of manufacturer, size, and style, BUY TWO PAIRS! Then alternate them between hikes. This may seem extravagant, but you've gotta believe me when I say it's tough to find ideal hiking boots for your feet.

*If you're deeply interested in the details of hiking boots, read the Ultimate Guide to boots on the HFH website.

BEST HIKING SHOES

When you're searching for a pair of hiking shoes, you want them to be reasonably priced, fast to lace and unlace, lightweight and responsive to trail conditions, comfortable from the first step due to the contours of the heel cup and mid-sole, able to withstand reasonable amounts of trail mud and moisture, protective of your toes, heel, arch and soles, as well as grippy on slick or inclined surfaces.

Whew! We're not asking for much, are we?!

The underlying qualities are exactly the same as for hiking boots: support, comfort and durability.

Your mission? To find hiking shoes that not only meet these criteria but also work well with the sizing peculiarities of your feet.

Sad, true fact: This might take some time, so be patient as you begin your quest for the best hiking shoes.

And beware of anyone who tells you that you've just gotta have a particular brand because "everyone" wears them on the trail! *Only your feet can decide what's an ideal fit.*

Shoes are a good way to go if you're not sure you'll be in this hiking thing for the long haul. You can always wear them for yard work, dog walking or other outdoor activities and still get your money's worth out of them.

The Resources section of Chapter One gives you a few ideas to consider if you're in the market for hiking shoes.

HIKING SOCKS

You probably haven't thought much about hiking socks, but now you need to start paying close attention to which socks work best with your chosen trail footwear.

It's not an overstatement to say that your feet are one of your most precious assets as a hiker. Together with your brain, they keep you safe and get you back to the trail head no matter what is going on around you.

To **thank your feet** for their endless duty on the trail, you must provide them with a great pair of hiking socks.

Notice the word "*hiking*" in front of the socks. You need socks that can stand up to the friction, heat, stress, and swollen feet generated by a hike.

Your $1 bargain bin specials won't cut it. Or will cut it for just long enough to usher you into the wonderful world of blisters (sarcasm intended).

Consider this sentence as your invitation to enter the ***wonderful universe of hiking socks***.

The universal fact is this: You need two pairs of socks if you wear hiking boots. And they need to be two different types.

What?? Two stinkin' pairs? (NOTE: They should NOT stink when you take them home from the store. That comes later.)

Yes, I kid you not. (If you're a hiking shoes devotee, skip this part because one pair of socks will suffice in most conditions.)

You need an inner and an outer pair to protect and work in unison with your feet in your hiking boots.

Inner pair: Sock liners, they're called. They have lots of responsibilities.

-They must conform to the contours of your foot and boot without sliding around.

-They should wick your sweat away from your skin, to prevent your epidermis from losing contact with your dermis (OUCH - a blister!).

-And they should make a reasonable attempt at absorbing foot odors. (Have you smelled your favorite pair of shoes lately? I'll be here when you come back.)

Outer pair: These are probably what you think about when you visualize "hiking" socks.

They come in all sorts of colors and varieties and price points, which makes sock shopping lots of fun. However, avoid getting sucked into *sock overload* by focusing on the main questions:

-Will they pad your heels and soles from the wear and tear created by putting all of your weight on your feet, hour after hour, day after day?

-Will they fit snugly over your liners, but not too snugly?

-Will the heels and toes *not* wear out after a few hikes?

Hiking socks will be labeled to indicate how much wear and tear they will stand up to, and how much cushioning to expect. Look for the words "*light*" or "*heavy*" or "*expedition*" or "*trekking*".

When you go sock shopping, recall these labels but also remember the features you are looking (and paying) for:

-cushioning,

-heel and toe reinforcement,

-moisture and heat control,

-comfort, and

-durability.

Personally, I choose the "*trekking*" variety because they're built to take what I dish out inside my boots. And even so, I replace my socks every other summer because the heels and toes wear out. So don't expect durability miracles!

And my apologies in advance for sticker shock. Activity specific socks might seem a bit overpriced, but go back to first principles: **Your feet qualify as your most important hiking gear**.

I beg you, skimp somewhere else if you have to, but never on your feet!

To achieve the ideal condition of liner socks playing nicely with outer socks, and both pairs playing nicely with your hiking footwear, you have to shop around a little for the right materials.

Nylon and spandex will ensure a well fitted shape. Merino wool has good moisture wicking properties. Polyester is sometimes blended in to enhance thermal regulation. You have lots of options, to say the least.

Tip: In hiking shoes or trail running shoes it's possible to get by on just one pair of socks.

Personally, I'm skeptical. I cherish my epidermis and dermis to a high degree, and will do anything it takes to keep them together (i.e. blister free feet).

If two pairs of socks seems like too much bulk, please try the combo at least once on a long-ish (over 5 miles) hike. This assumes that you have trail footwear that can accommodate the thickness of the socks.

That's why it's a great idea to shop for socks first, followed by the footwear.

And don't forget to bring your chosen hiking socks to your boot-buying expedition at a local gear store. (If you're really lucky, the store will have a "borrow" bin of socks if you forget.)

DAYHIKE BACKPACKS

Choosing a backpack is both an art and a science, involving some issues you probably haven't run into before: ergonomics, lightweight yet durable materials such as denier nylon, adjustable waist belts, sternum straps and ventilation designs.

Here's a fun fact behind that list: Backpack manufacturers pride themselves on little twists and improvements on basic designs, making their product line into unique backpacks with deep brand loyalty.

But a backpack is pretty much a backpack at heart. So before you become brand loyal, become knowledgeable about how to choose a backpack.

To help you, here are general Backpacks 101 tips, regardless of manufacturer. If you implement these tips, you'll know exactly which pack, waiting for you amongst all of the hiking packs in the backpack store, is perfect for your unique hiking plans.

1. Decide whether quality or price is most important to you. There are plenty of cheap backpacks you can get at least one season out of, and that's a fact.

But if you're going to be in this hiking thing for the long haul (small backpack joke) you should buy the highest quality pack possible.

It will provide more comfort on the trail, and be less of a financial drain on your long term hiking budget.

2. If you're just starting out as a hiker, **don't look at customized backpacks**. They have a mind numbing array of custom features and while they literally fit you like a glove, they are murderously expensive.

There's also a whiff of "look how cool I am" attached to having a hand made custom pack, which might not be worth the extra money.

As a dayhiker, you need a **basic pack to start with**, and can work your way up to one of these customized beauties over time if you so desire.

3. It's easy to **fall victim to "buyer's fatigue"** unless you **do your homework ahead of time.**

-Go to the store (virtual or real) armed with a **short list of packs** to try on: brand, size (in liters), and the exact model you want to try on (see below).

-A phone call ahead of time saves you the heartache of arriving at a store only to hear "We just sold out of those." Ditto for shopping early during online sales.

-Arrange your schedule so you have plenty of time. You don't want to rush to judgment because it's closing time, or you have to catch a train.

-Eat and drink something (see Chapter 3) before you start shopping. A dehydration headache or hypoglycemic brain fog will lead you into some bad decisions. (This advice also applies to hiking. And online dating, but that's a different book.)

4. Never trap yourself into the **"gotta have it" corner**.

If you have a hike coming up on the calendar, start right now to create that short list. You don't want to get stuck buying a less than ideal pack because you ran out of time.

This is especially true once you go looking for backpacking packs, which you will if the dayhiking bug progresses to its logical conclusion.

And I predict that if you get bitten by the dayhiking bug, it will explode into a backpacking fever requiring heavier gear. This is not lethal, just more expensive.

If you want to look at bigger backpacking packs while you're at it, be sure to read the backpacking gear tips on the HFH website first.

How To Size Up Backpacks

Now for some specific tips to find the pack of your dreams, or at least one that won't fight you on the trail.

Size: Reasonable choices for daypacks wander between 36 liters and 24 liters, unless you want to go super light and carry almost nothing. Read Chapter 2 (Ten Essentials) before making that drastic decision.

Sizing also brings up the issue of torso length. Two ways to go here: Find a pack with shorter or longer torso lengths, or one that is adjustable through a wide range.

This is especially important if you are dayhiking for weight loss. As your dimensions change, the pack will accommodate you without having to be replaced.

Ventilation: A pack with a mesh "wall" and plenty of airspace between your sweaty shirt and the pack itself is ideal.

In cold weather you can stash an extra fleece or jacket there to prevent cool breezes, but realize that you'll probably overheat even in cold weather if your pace is fast enough (Chapter 8).

Zippers: These should be equipped with fabric pulls that are long enough to be grasped easily, enabling you to open them one handed or wearing gloves.

Zippers should be longer than they need to be, meaning that you can get your whole hand and arm in the compartment if necessary.

And they should slide easily even under gritty conditions. Plastic is lighter than metal, and is the zipper standard on today's packs because they don't rust or jam easily.

Compartments: How many is too many? Too few? That depends on how many items you'll be carrying on your hike, including the Ten Essentials (good old Chapter 2 again).

A small daypack should have at least 2 compartments, one right at the top to catch all the little-but-significant stuff a dayhiker needs, and a large one that's easy to get into during rest stops.

Some of the packs on the larger end of the size scale divide the large compartment with a removable fabric divider, creating a bottom area that is accessed with its own zipper.

If you use a hydration system (Chapter 4), there should be dedicated space inside the pack to accommodate a full water bladder. Also look for the hole where the tubing from the bladder exits the pack at one of the top corners.

Extra pockets (usually small and zippered) on the hip belt or straps are convenient for stashing sunscreen, snacks, lip balm, and other odds and ends in an easy to get to place. But they're not compartments which are essential to your success on the trail.

Hip/waist belt: You need this belt to secure the pack to your body and to transfer weight from your spinal column to your hip bones, through your legs and into your feet.

Look for a belt that is well padded, not too wide, with strap adjustments to accommodate bulky layering. The belt should close easily (snap together) with a lightweight yet sturdy plastic buckle which can be replaced if damaged or lost.

Hip belts are one feature that distinguish various price points on a day pack. The less padding, the cheaper the price.

But remember that your comfort is priceless on the trail.

Tapered shoulder harness: Who needs really wide gizmos on a day pack? Not humans with breast tissue!

The shoulder harness should have contoured padded straps and a sternum buckle on a strap to secure your load and transfer weight away from your fragile shoulder girdle.

Sternum is just another way to say chest, by the way.

Mesh side pockets: Look for at least one, for your water bottle(s), unused hiking poles, and maps. If you have a hydration bladder tucked safely into your pack, and you don't use trekking poles, maybe you don't need side pockets.

Bonus features: Small mesh hip belt pockets to stash trail treats and lip balm are nice, but not strictly necessary unless you're a lip balm addict.

A rain cover that tucks up into the bottom of the pack in a zippered compartment is nice in certain climates.

A color that doesn't make you queasy is always welcome (brief pause for rant against little girl pink hiking gear; apologies if you absolutely love pink; okay, all done now).

Price: A reasonable price point for a day pack is somewhere around $100.

For that amount of money you should get high quality stitching, durable materials like Denier nylon, (higher numbers are tougher, but also heavier), lightweight quick release buckles, tough straps and belts with double stitching at ends to prevent unraveling, and easy to use zippers.

DAY HIKE CLOTHING

You can use whatever clothing is hanging in your closet as you hit the trail for the first few times.

Or you can commit to purchasing athletic clothing suitable for daily walks, a gym workout, dayhikes or the best of all 3 healthy habits.

Let's take a peek at the basic foundational items: your sports bra and underwear. Then we'll build you a trail wardrobe you can rely on in all kinds of weather.

Sports bras: Comfort if not modesty dictates some sort of sports bra for hiking.

What you put next to your skin matters on a hike. You want your sweat to be wicked away so you don't feel clammy and wet.

You want your body odors to be minimized.

And you want to look good.

This foundation layer can't be too bulky because you'll be layering more on top of it, even in warm weather.

And don't forget about softness and the need to minimize any chance of nipple and armpit chafing.

In a hurry? Hop onto the HFH website and read about features in good hiking sports bras.

Stick with me here for the basics.

There are two basic approaches to keeping your chest under wraps during a day hike: a shelf bra and a cup bra.

Shelf bras don't always provide the support you might need/want. Factor in how much sweat you'll produce, and calculate your tolerance for it pooling between your "uni-boob" shelf.

You might also find nipple chafing a serious problem with a flimsy shelf sports bra. (If you've never experienced chafing on this part of your body, you might scoff at the idea – but it's not a fun thing for a hiker to experience, and it takes forever to heal.)

A built-in cup sports bra is definitely more comfortable if you want to avoid the bounce and the sweaty "stuck-together" side effect of hard trail work. It gives you a more natural appearance in photographs (if that's important to you), and evenly distributes the front load across your shoulders and back.

Heads up: You will have to try on *many* brands until you find the one with the magical combination of fit, form and function.

Once you do, buy several and rotate them through your hiking clothing line up. Your sweat combined with trail dirt eats into their life span, as does frequent wash/dry cycles.

What about under wire bras? I hope you're not surprised to hear that you should leave them at home! They will pinch and bind you, and you don't want to be wearing metal during a thunderstorm. True story!

How to find the right sports bra

You might already know that sports bras are available in a dizzying array of fabrics, styles and colors. But here are a few pivotal questions to ponder when selecting a sports bra to ensure that it becomes one of your favorite pieces of hiking apparel.

Will this bra be easy to get off once I'm sweaty and hot? Racer back -vs- standard back styles will perform differently.

Pull on styles tend to lead to a wrestling match with yourself, compared to the hook-and-eye styles.

If the straps are adjusted with Velcro, they can be released quickly to help you exit the bra or make adjustments while hiking.

How much support do I need? Level trail walking doesn't lend itself to much bounce, but if you're losing lots of elevation during your hike you might need a built-in cup design to keep from jostling your girls.

Tip: Your daypack's sternum strap (which buckles across your chest above your nipples; see above) will provide a bit of support as you move.

Even if you tend toward not much going on up top, I'd recommend a base layer anyway, to protect your nipples from chafing or your pack from rubbing your back raw. And lucky you - you won't need a ton of support built in, which means your sports bra can be lighter weight and will dry faster once it soaks up your sweat.

Is this fabric moisture wicking, odor absorbent and fast drying?
If you have a low tolerance for sweat, you'll want to buy a sports bra made with antimicrobial and proven moisture wicking fabrics such as polypropylene.

On the other hand, if you're going to throw the bra into the washing machine right after each hike, maybe you don't need to go all out on this feature.

Note that cotton will absorb your sweat easily & wick it away from your skin, but will not release the moisture quickly, leaving you with a wet soggy under layer that is unpleasant and potentially dangerous on cold days.

One final caveat: This area of your body is highly personal. It might take a few tries before you find the right amount of snugness, support, ease of removal, wicking and fabric thickness which suits you best for dayhiking.

Experiment until you get it just right. And please take my advice: buy a few when you find just the right style.

How To Choose Hiking Underwear

Again, we're in highly individual territory.

Here's my preference: I like **slippery fabric** such as nylon blends because they play well with my hiking pants when I clamber over logs or stride uphill.

A cotton panel in the crotch feels soft and helps draw moisture away. This is important to avoid infections if you're prone to them. I realize that violates the "cotton kills" athletic clothing rule, but it's a small amount and right up against an endless source of body heat, so no worries.

Don't expect underwear made completely of cotton to dry quickly after a summer shower or a dip in that beckoning alpine lake. If you've never experienced the joy of hiking in cold wet cotton underwear, consider yourself warned.

Also pay attention to the cut of the underwear. Low cuts (especially thongs) may be too skimpy to prevent chafing from your pants rubbing against your pack. And thongs tend to migrate into the middle, making you walk differently.

High waisted underwear may be too binding around your waist, if you already have a backpack strap and a camera strap around you. High waists also trap more heat and sweat against your skin.

For these reasons I recommend that you aim for a *mid rise cut* which covers you enough to prevent chafing, and is slippery enough to move with you during your hike. See Chapter One Resources for a few ideas.

As with sports bras, it may take a few tries before you find the magical base layer. And you may need several types for seasonal and activity level gradations.

Once you find a pair that works well, buy several pairs because believe it or not, underwear manufacturers have yearly models just like car companies! Don't be disappointed when you try to find "THE PAIR" in a few years, only to have your heart broken (words of wisdom, earned the hard way).

JACKETS

The best hiking jacket is the one that fits your body and your budget without causing strain. Duh! Easy words to say, but hard to find that perfect jacket for your hiking adventures.

If you're just starting out as a hiker, don't spend a lot of money on trail jackets until you've decided which type of terrain and climate you want to explore.

It's quite easy to over-buy a jacket, because they are loaded with ventilation and adjustment features that you'll never use on mild summer days.

Tip: Look for **versatility** and **durability.** These 2 attributes are worth the money, every time. If you can wear the jacket around town, in the garden, on your next plane trip AND on the trail, good deal!

Bringing a jacket on every day hike is a good habit. If you've chosen a decent sized day pack, you will have plenty of room for a rolled up jacket.

Never make the rookie mistake of starting off on a fine sunny morning in short sleeves, only to end up a chilled, shivering hiker with no jacket when the thunderstorm rolls in (there's that darned Chapter 2 Ten Essentials thing again).

How To Choose A Hiking Jacket

The first thing to consider is how many layers you'll be wearing beneath the jacket.

While you're on the trail you'll be working up a sweat, and maintaining a higher body temperature than if you were lounging around at base camp. So choose a jacket that accommodates the number of layers you'll be using.

Over your sports bra and underwear (your base layer) you'll be wearing a lightweight, fitted hiking shirt. (mid layer). Over that will go your jacket (outer layer) if it's a breezy day or you get caught in the rain.

A thin windbreaker or fleece pullover will keep your body heat trapped against your skin. But you might want a more fitted jacket to prevent wind and rain from blowing up your backside in wilder weather, or when hiking through rough and/or wet vegetation.

Planning a dayhike in cool and wet conditions? You need a looser jacket to go over your long sleeved shirt and vest: layering without hindering your movements is your aim.

Look for "**jacket optimization features**" like cinching, removable or fold-away hood, zippered pockets and removable liner so you can get the most out of the jacket. These versatile jackets cost more, but provide more value on the trail.

Do you need a hood for day hikes?My recommendation is to always purchase a jacket with a hood, but look for an option to tuck the hood away in a flat zippered pouch at the neckline. This gives you the best of both worlds!

A **hood** can be pulled up on top of a hat to provide an additional layer of warmth, or can keep wind and rain off your neck and head if you've forgotten your hat. It can also shield your identity if you meet someone you'd rather not greet on the trail.

Which jacket length is best for you? That depends.

Hip length will keep you drier, but will ride up a bit from the motion of your pack. A **shorter jacket** gives no protection from cold rocks or wet logs when you sit down for a snack, but you will find them less binding and therefore desirable in better weather.

Some jackets are **tapered**, longer in back than front. If a hip length jacket pulls against your thighs, look for one with a tapered fit to get protection from rain and damp ground without giving up mobility.

The higher the price point, the more likely it is to expect the**fabrics** to keep you warm and dry, regardless of the amount of wind, rain and snow coming at you. Also look for taped seams, waterproof zippers, and an overhang on the hood to keep water off your body.

Again, expect to pay for the high quality fabrics which are breathable while repelling moisture. You want your body heat to dissipate without creating an internal rain shower.

You will come to cherish a jacket with the ability to make adjustments at the neck and cuffs, dictated by weather conditions and your internal temperature fluctuations.

Jacket fabrics should also bend and twist easily with you and create minimal noise, although there are degrees of success depending upon which blend of fabrics is used. Nothing is more irritating than hiking in a sea of noise created by your own jacket.

On higher price point jackets, all points of excessive wear should be **reinforced**, meaning the life span of this jacket is extended. Usually, this means wrists and elbows, although the abrasion of your pack could also thin out the fabric at the shoulder areas.

Zippers are really important. You want an easy up and down central zipper that won't get stuck or jammed when it's cold and wet and your fingers get clumsy. Two way motion is a great feature to make adjustments in the field, or to un-jam a stuck zipper.

Zippers on pockets need to be durable and easy to access even when wearing gloves. These are usually the first zippers to succumb to overuse, so having Velcro reinforcement is a nice touch for pockets.

However, while **Velcro closures** are reliable, they attract stray string, fuzz and trail detritus, hindering their ability to grip tightly. They are also noisy, which might be a problem if you're nature watching or sneaking up on a trail buddy.

And **forget buttons**. They have a tendency to fall off just when you need them most. They're also hard to deal with when your fingers are cold and wet.

On a more expensive jacket, you also want to find **vents**, created by zippers in your armpit and chest areas to allow body heat and moisture to escape. It's great to be able to regulate your body heat without removing the jacket, especially on rainy days.

That covers all of the features to watch for on a hiking jacket.

Now here's my philosophy on hiking jackets: When my life does not literally depend on my jacket, I wear less expensive brands. I know that I won't get the same level of performance and durability, and I'm okay with that. I also don't cringe when I fall in the mud or snag myself on trail debris.

But when I'm going to be out in unpredictable weather or on rugged terrain, I wear my top quality jacket. I rely upon its design features (outlined above) to protect my body heat and keep me as dry as possible.

Here are some options for **choosing jackets for dayhiking**.

Maybe you already have a jacket hanging in the closet. If it's cotton, don't consider it for day hiking. Cotton does a good job of wicking sweat away from your body in hot weather, but not dissipating it (along with associated odors).

And in cold wet conditions, cotton will set you up for hypothermia (decreased core temperature).

The least expensive way to go is to wear a nylon lightweight jacket. Nylon does snag on branches, and it's not weather proof, but if you snag or rip this jacket, you won't be out a lot of money. And don't forget, duct tape fixes everything!

A soft shell jacket is a good choice for mild weather, packs down small and generally keeps cool breezes and mist at bay. It's an option for fall and spring hikes when light rainfall is expected.

Are expensive hiking jackets worth the money? Great question. No easy answers. Go back to the quality versus functionality conundrum.

Quality is synonymous with names like North Face, Arc'teryx, Patagonia and Helly Hansen, just to name a few of the brands I've invested in when shopping for weatherproof hiking clothing.

These jackets are engineered (some might say over-engineered) to deliver weatherproof, easy to use features that make wet, cold weather easier to deal with. But you're going to pay for all of that.

The trick to avoiding sticker shock? Shop at the end of the season to scoop up deals. You'd be surprised how much of a discount you can score with a little detective work.

Another way to look at this is in terms of investing in your safety, comfort and well being.

I've paid full price for two hiking jackets many years ago, and am still wearing them for extreme hiking adventures in Greenland and Alaska. There have been times, shivering in my tent as the wind pounded sleet overhead, when I was extremely grateful for wearing a jacket that got me safely into that tent.

A third way? Ask for these jackets as gifts! I'm sure someone in your life would love to watch your eyes light up when one of the best hiking jackets lands in your lap.

HATS

Believe it when I tell you that hats have a lot to do with the enjoyment of your hike.

The right hat will shade your eyes, protect your head against bushes and dive bombing birds (no joke! owls in particular), hold your hair off your sweaty neck, mop up sweat before it runs into your eyes (along with sunscreen – OUCH!), shield your face from excessive UV radiation exposure, and shield your identity if you meet someone on the trail you'd rather not speak with (ex-boyfriends, perhaps?).

When you hike in less than ideal conditions, you'll need to keep your head and ears covered to preserve body heat. Too much heat is lost in these areas for you to be comfortable, let alone safe, going bare headed.

Hats are extremely important during sunny hot weather, too. Create your own shade, and keep UV radiation from the sun off your skin, with the right hat. This is smart for cutting down on water loss but also protects you from premature wrinkles and skin cancer concerns.

A **ball cap style** of hat is a good choice for cutting glare and shading the top of your head. Be sure it's vented if you'll be wearing it when it's hot or if the trail breaks out of the dense forest to cross open slopes.

Warning: You'll end up collecting several different weights in different colors, to match the different seasons. Don't fight it. It's all part of falling in love with the trail.

Tip: Don't use ball caps with Velcro closures. They catch on your hair, making them painful to adjust. Also, Velcro accumulates trail debris and stray threads or fuzz from your collar - yuck.

A **sun hat** will need a wide brim, and may have a cord to cinch under your chin when the wind comes up.

Again, be sure it's vented so you don't cook the top of your head.

Tip: Be sure the back of the hat's brim doesn't collide with the top of your backpack. A too-wide brim hitting your pack interferes with your vision of the trail, and may result in cuss words being shared with innocent bystanders like trees and squirrels.

A **beanie style** hat will give you ear coverage. A hat with ear flaps goes one better, but also muffles sound which can be important if you're listening for environmental cues such as a waterfall.

If you're going to be hiking when it's really windy and/or cold, invest in a **balaclava**. This is a hat and neck scarf all in one.

I recommend including it in your ten essentials (Chapter 2) as a vital piece of extra clothing. You can also sit on it, wrap an injured body area in it, and use it to store trail specimens like pine cones or mushrooms.

Tip: Carry a balaclava year round, at the bottom of your pack. One never knows!

Another thing about hats: They reveal a hiker's trail personality.

No, really!

Play a little game with yourself on your next hike: Focus on the head wear of oncoming hikers, rather than their faces, gender or age. What clues do you pick up about them?

Great conversation starters, too. "Hey! When were you in Yellowstone?"

TREKKING POLES

Some hikers will tell you that trekking or hiking poles are optional. Don't believe them!

Poles are used by day hikers in a variety of ways to:

-improve **balance** on steep slopes,

-provide **confidence** while negotiating slick trails or tricky stream crossings,

-probe ahead to **safely cross** a snow bridge or fast flowing stream,

-**fend off** aggressive dogs on the trail when the owners are nowhere in sight,

-take a load off **knees** while hiking downhill,

-double as **emergency shelter supports** if you need to make camp overnight,

-provide a nice **upper body workout**,

-click against rocks to **alert your hiking buddies of your location**, and

-**collapse** into a small footprint to ride along in a day pack until they're needed.

Research has shown that **hiking with poles can increase the number of calories burned**, without making you feel more tired. That's useful when hiking for weight control or weight loss, right?

It will also motivate you to **try longer hikes** as you get hooked on dayhiking.

Using poles will cause your heart to pump harder to support the increased oxygen demand from your arm muscles. This gives you a **stronger heart muscle** without increasing your pace or tackling harder terrain.

One more plus: Your leg muscles don't have to work as hard when you use trekking poles, because they provoke a longer stride length as you lean out over them.

This means you **cover more ground per step** but not at the expense of more muscle contractions. You'll have energy left at the end of the day to chow down on a delicious post-hike dinner.

And there's a uniquely female reason for using poles on a dayhike: our hip and knee anatomy. Female hikers have wider pelvic basins and a different angle between hips and knee than male hikers. Using **poles protects the knees from sudden twists** during a stumble by transferring force away from bony structures.

Post-puberty but not yet menopausal females (teens through forties) also have fluctuating hormone levels during their monthly cycles, making ligaments more prone to tearing or stretching at certain times of the month. Hiking poles **give extra support** while striding and negotiating steep terrain during these more vulnerable days.

See? You really should consider poles as essential hiking gear.

Features of good hiking poles

If you're looking for the perfect trekking poles, you've got to be sure they will fit your hands without causing fatigue as you swing them. That's why you need to buy hiking poles specifically made for women.

This is especially true for petite women, who need shorter poles and smaller hand grips.

Be sure to try the poles in the store, swinging your arms and pumping them up and down to simulate trail conditions. Ignore the funny looks, it's for a good cause: your comfort on the trail.

Features you absolutely need to pay attention to when shopping for poles:

-They must be **adjustable** so you can shorten/lengthen them according to trail conditions, and so you can **collapse them** to their smallest height to stow in your pack.

-They should be as **lightweight** as you can afford (preferably under one pound). Carbon fiber is the lightest, most expensive, and most prone to breakage under a heavy load. Aluminum is also a light choice and you'd be hard pressed to break an aluminum trekking pole - although you can bend it if you really try.

-If your knees or hips are at all cranky about hill walking, purchase poles with **shock absorbing internal springs** to take some of the punch out of your steep descents.

-There are several types of **locking mechanisms** to choose from to keep your poles from collapsing when you put weight on them, and I've used all of them: twist lock, button, external latch/lever/clamp, and a combo of twist and lever.

Currently I'm using the "clamp it down tight" type of lock. I appreciate how rock solid that feels.

-**Hand grip** materials: I've used cork, foam and rubber (recommended only in winter). Cork comes out a winner in my book, because it doesn't slip around in my sweaty palms.

Hard foam is also a great choice, and doesn't absorb sweat as readily as cork.

-If you're going to use the trekking poles for **winter hiking and/or snowshoeing**, you'll need to be able to swap out the small **baskets** on the end of the poles for something larger so the poles don't sink with each step.

Tip: Be sure you can get the baskets off and on easily, and that you can buy replacement baskets if you lose one in the snow.

-**Pole tip** materials: Rubber tips fit over carbide tips to give you a wide range of options for traction. If you break off a tip, you can buy replacement tips that install easily. If you use your poles for daily training walks around the neighborhood, putting the rubber tips on will extend the life of the carbide tips.

-**Wrist straps** are handy while on slopes to ensure you don't lose your pole if you lose your grip. Sometimes I give my hands a rest and allow the poles to dangle for a few steps. And the straps have saved me from having to down-climb to retrieve a pole that got away.

There are many **price points for trekking poles**, reflecting all of the above features. Pick your top 3 "must have" features, and see what you will have to pay for a good set of hiking poles. Don't be afraid to invest in poles, because of all of the reasons I've shared above.

Not ready to buy a pair? **Rent or borrow** some, and note how you feel using them on the trail, as well as the next day.

Chapter One Summed Up

In this first chapter, a lot of ground was covered.

That's because you plan to cover a lot of ground, and I want you to be as comfortable and prepared as possible.

Don't try to absorb everything all at once.

Select one piece of gear, re-read the tips, and commit to a shopping trip for just that one item.

Learn as you go - which stores, which sales people, which brands suit you best? Keep notes!

Did this whirlwind tour through the gear essentials for dayhiking leave you dizzy?

Never fear, the Chapter One Resources are here. It's your chance to take a close look at the gear I use every day, and that's why I feel good about recommending it to you.

And don't forget, you can send me an email and get your specific question answered quickly.

Chapter One Take-Aways

Don't be defeated by your feet. **Choose the right trail footwear** for your type of dayhiking after you decide where you want to hike (Chapter 5).

Your choice of hiking socks is every bit as important as your footwear. **Socks and footwear are a dynamic, mighty hiking duo**.

Choose a hiking daypack that gives you the right volume, fit and features while delivering durability and style for your chosen price point.

Hiking clothing should be protective, moisture wicking, odor resistant, fast drying and comfortable. And if you're a trail fashionista, it should look good, too.

Trekking poles provide stability and help with balance, but most importantly they direct forces away from your precious knee and hip joints. Investing in a pair of poles will pay dividends years later on the trail.

The **Resource section** at the end of every chapter, including this one, will give you even more recommendations and information.

Chapter One Resources

Hiking For Her Gear Recommendations

It pays to be selective about the brands you use, and the places you shop.

But where do you start?

Right here, at Hiking For Her!

After 4+ decades of purchasing hiking gear, I have a pretty good handle on how (and where) to gear shop.

Tip: Be sure to sink into the technical details, manufacturer's specifications, and posted reviews to get a well rounded view of every piece of hiking gear. The more data you have, the more informed gear buying decisions you will make.

FOOTWEAR RECOMMENDATIONS

Lightweight hiking boots: I love my Keens! Light on the feet, no break in time, reasonably weather proof, moderate durability, a great price for the quality, and did I mention they feel great?

Heavy duty leather boots: I love the heavy leather boots I learned to backpack in, and was reluctant to switch to lightweight options. But my Keen enthusiasm is rather apparent, don't you think?

However, I do wear heavy leather boots for certain types of hiking. You will want to consider them, too, if you:

-hike on rocky, unstable footing.

-want full ankle support and protection.

-love how rock solid a heavy Vibram or rubber blend sole feels.

-will someday be carrying a heavy load for long distances, as in an extended backpacking trip with limited resupply options.

Zamberlan, Alico and other hand made boots from Europe are worth a look (and the investment price tag, for serious hikers).

Hiking shoes: Read about the Salomons I use by searching for my review on the HFH website.

Trail sandals are not recommended except for stream crossings. If you're going to cross water above your ankles, consider using sandals rather than subjecting your boots to all of that water.

Sandals also spare the bottoms of your tender feet.

It comes down to safety - can you make it across without losing your footing in sandals? If not, keep your boots on, but take some care in drying them out later.

I can't live without my Teva sandals, and you will find them on my feet both on and off the trail. They're sporty looking and solid, that's for sure!

Winter hiking boots (snowshoeing):

I grew up in a snowy, cold upper Michigan town, so I know winter boots inside and out. The brand I come back to year after year is Sorel.

These boots may seem overbuilt, but in fact, every feature is incredibly useful and well designed. And who doesn't love the security of triple stitching?

Rest assured, you'll like the way they perform on the trail, or attached to your snowshoes.

Here's a company that also knows winter conditions: The Getzs company was founded in Marquette MI (just a few miles as the crow flies from my home town).

I have great respect for this company, because it doesn't mess around with trendy stuff. Getzs sticks to the basics, and does them well. So it's no surprise that they feature Sorel winter boots.

You can take a look at all of my winter boot recommendations, including Sorels, on the HFH website.

Quality may seem like an steep investment up front, but it pays dividends over the years. You will never have to worry about the condition of your feet in Sorel boots.

Note that I've had the same pair for over 15 years! Not even kidding, fifteen years of keeping my feet warm and dry. (The Sorel brand has been purchased by a different company, so it's possible that branding and quality changes may occur. Read current reviews carefully.)

SOCK RECOMMENDATIONS

I am a loyal fan of the brands which have served me well over the years. I humbly offer them as a place to start, if you don't have any sock lending buddies to turn to for advice.

Read all of my hiking sock tips on the HFH website, and pick a pair to try.

You'll see that I prefer Dry CoolMax Liner Socks, and Thorlo or Smart Wool outer socks.

Lightweight Thorlos are a good choice for moderate dayhiking.

As are SmartWool medium weight women's crew hiking socks.

And if you're plagued by blisters, Armaskin and Injinji anti-blister socks are worth a close look.

DAYPACK RECOMMENDATIONS

What I use: Osprey and Deuter.

The website will give you all the details if you use those brand names to search for my reviews.

SPORTS BRA RECOMMENDATIONS

To get good performance out of a sports bra, avoid the cheapie versions that give little to no support and wear out after a few months of soaking up sweat.

You want to do business with companies that really know how to build a sports bra. There are 2 companies that I use over and over again, and have no hesitation recommending to you.

Moving Comfort (exactly the right name for hikers!) has lots of options, allowing you to pick a bra that accommodates your cup size along with modesty and support preferences.

The style I prefer for hiking is easy to get in and out of, it has adequate support and full coverage, and the straps are wide enough to protect my shoulders from pack abrasion.

The Moving Comfort brand name was acquired by Brooks, so read current reviews carefully for quality and performance changes.

Title Nine (a reference to legally mandated inclusive policies for women's sports in the U.S.) provides great "how to buy a sports bra" tutorials. Their clever punning (much better than mine; "bust musts", for example) is entertaining and takes the edge off what could be a struggle to find the perfect hiking sports bra. It might take a few tries to find exactly the bra you need, but they certainly make it easy!

Need plus size sports bras? Visit the HFH website's recommendations for getting a great fit as well as high performance.

UNDERWEAR RECOMMENDATIONS

To read about my current favorites, you know where to go!

Note that I prefer mid cuts, made of a wicking, slippery fabric.

JACKET RECOMMENDATIONS

When my life does not literally depend on my jacket, I wear less expensive brands. I know that I won't get the same level of performance and durability, and I'm okay with that.

For beginning hikers, look for fit and function, along with low price point.

Typically, that means a nylon jacket with a hood, and pit vents if you pay a little more.

However, lightweight nylon is not heavy duty so shouldn't be put in extreme conditions and expected to perform well over long periods of time.

But if you rip it, it's easy to replace.

While you're on the trail you'll be working up a sweat, thus maintaining a higher body temperature than if you were lounging around at the trail head. Choose a jacket that accommodates the number of layers you'll be using, and realize that not every hiker will want to wear numerous layers.

In fact, you might want a more fitted jacket to prevent wind and rain from blowing up your backside.

Read why I love my Arcteryx jacket, a fairly roomy shell, allowing for layers beneath it without hindering your movements, by visiting the Hiking Jackets page on the website.

This company, renowned for its quality jackets, also makes more form fitting versions. If you want the best jacket possible, take a hard look at this company.

HAT RECOMMENDATIONS

I have a full repertoire of hiking hats. The website page on Hiking Hats will give you a peek at my hiking hat collection, and explain why you should probably start your hat collection soon.

Styles to consider:

-beanies;

-ball baps;

-balaclava;

-sun hats.

A great approach for sun protection is to wear a hat that protects your face and neck from the sun's rays, while giving good ventilation and the option of tossing it in the washing machine at the end of the hike.

I also recommend a neck gaiter. It can be used on your head or neck in many different ways, giving you versatility as well as warmth.

And of course, there are always ear muffs and head bands. I've got quite a collection, and you will, too, once you see how functional and lightweight they are. Great for daily training walks around home or at the dog park, too.

POLE RECOMMENDATIONS

I've owned 4 brands of hiking poles over the years: REI, Komperdell, Black Diamond and Leki.

I've used Black Diamond poles exclusively over the past four years (hiking in all 4 seasons in varied terrain), and they've taken everything I've dished out.

Hiking For Her's Additional Information

Pop these key words into the search box on the website for a ton of details about each topic.

Hiking boots

Hiking shoes

Hiking jackets

Hiking socks

Gear reviews

Hiking clothing layering system

Boot lacing tips

If you still have numerous questions, or need some assistance (or a pep talk) for choosing the best hiking gear for your dayhiking adventures, I've got an easy, fun solution.

Schedule a gear chat with Diane!

That's right, you and I can chat on the phone, for whatever length of time works for you. Call it "virtual gear shopping." Read all of the details on the Gear Chat page of the HFH website.

And if you happen to live in the Seattle area, we can do the same thing at the gear store of your choice.

Retail therapy for hikers, what's not to love?

Chapter 2: The Ten Essentials

It's essential to stay warm, dry, and able to take care of yourself, should you need to spend the night outdoors or respond to a trail emergency.

That just makes sense, right?

In this chapter, you'll meet the famous Hiking **Ten Essentials** and find answers to these questions:

-What are they?

-Why are they essential?

-Why should we add female hiking intuition to the list?

THE FAMOUS LIST: HIKING TEN ESSENTIALS

Don't be caught without these hiking ten essentials in your pack (unless you want your Professional Hiker card to be revoked).

Seriously, on every day hike, what's in your pack must provide you with what you need to keep safe, sane, and "unlost" under any weather conditions. Leave these items behind at your own peril:

1. Extra food and water

2. Extra clothing

3. Sunglasses

4. Knife

5. Fire starter

6. Matches

7. First aid supplies

8. Flashlight

9. Map(s)

10. Compass

All of these essentials are *common sense*, right? Don't forget to pack that, too.

Your brain is a major asset when you run into trouble and have to use your ten essentials.

A calm, matter of fact approach to trail trouble (a.k.a. common sense), coupled with your ten essentials, are going to pull you through whatever the trail throws at you.

Convinced you'll never run into trouble? I sincerely hope you're correct, but there's no way to know that for sure. These ten essentials stack the deck in your favor.

But let's pause for a brief reality check. Did you notice the big assumptions behind this list? Whoever first created it (a name lost to the mists of time) made some big assumptions about you.

Like what? Like you're already wearing the right clothing (Chapter 1), that you know how to use a map and compass (Chapter 7), you can deploy whatever is in your first aid kit, and that you will have fuel nearby to start and maintain a fire.

Those are not trivial assumptions! And they make reading the rest of this book mandatory, before you even begin to gather together these ten essentials.

Maybe the word "mandatory" got your attention. Good! Not to get all heavy on you, but your safety is your responsibility once you step onto a hiking trail.

Hopefully, you'll agree that Chapter 2 is a worthwhile investment of your time. Careful planning and attention to detail are traits of a strong dayhiker. So let's tackle this essential chapter to make you as strong as you can be.

Ten Essentials Close Up

"Essential" implies you gotta have it on the trail. Oh, so true!

Here's the common sense logic behind each of the hiking ten essentials that you will carry on every hike.

1. **FOOD**: **Extra food** is defined as over and above what you consider normal amounts of trail food (see Chapter 3).

On a day hike, a few trail snacks and lunch are going to fuel your hiking efforts. It won't cost you much in terms of weight or effort to throw in a few extra ounces of trail mix, or an extra energy bar, right?

Keep this in mind as you begin to plan your trail menu.

For carrying **extra water,** couple personal judgment with climate. You might want to monitor your daily water intake at home, and on your first few hikes. Do you seem unusually thirsty compared with other people? Then carry more water than your trail buddies.

Tip: Always know where surface water sources are located (see Chapter 5) just in case you have to refill a water bottle during an unexpected overnight stay.

2. **CLOTHING**: Flash forward in your mind beyond ideal warm, sunny conditions on the trail. What would nightfall in the forest/desert/river valley feel like?

Even though you have no intention of ever finding out, a few **extra layers** in your pack will give you a smart margin of safety.

Today's fleece and microfiber clothing is so lightweight, you have no excuse for *not* having an extra layer along - even in the height of summer.

Which layers make sense? Think about the areas of your body that lose heat quickly: head, face, hands, feet.

You can quickly don a lightweight fleece beanie and fleece gloves to trap your body heat. A neck gaiter or scarf can be pulled up around your nose and mouth to keep you cozy until you can get back to the trail head. And a jacket will help keep your core temperature within normal range after sundown.

It's probably overkill, but I recommend a pair of light weight rain pants tucked into the bottom of your pack year round, as an extra layer to ward off chills or damp ground.

And a pair of dry warm socks – priceless!

3. **SUNGLASSES**: Your eyes are a navigational tool. If you can't see, you are literally going nowhere.

That means you will have to rely upon the people back home to find you (you did leave an itinerary, or at least the name of the trail you're on with someone you trust, didn't you? See Chapter 5).

If there is snow travel involved in your plans, sunglasses shield your eyes from the UV rays bouncing merrily up from the snow surface into your eyeballs (you don't want to experience snow blindness, trust me on that one).

You might need extra protection if your eyes are lightly pigmented: glacier glasses for optimal protection against UV radiation, or sunglasses over your sunglasses, even on a dayhike.

Add sunscreen here, too. The short term effects of sunburned skin are dehydration and pain, again leading to impaired judgment. Carry SPF30 or higher, and stop at least twice on a hike to reapply it.

Formulas that promise to be "sweat proof" might linger a bit longer, but reapply at least once just to be safe during a long dayhike.

Caution! Sunscreen stings like crazy when it drips into your eyes, so wear a bandanna or hat with a moisture absorbent band to prevent this unpleasant side effect of doing the right thing.

4. **KNIFE**: A **knife** is just a way of saying "have something with a sharp edge" in case you have to whittle tree bark to start a fire, or gut a fish or frog in a survival situation.

I carry a Swiss Army knife that I rarely use, but the few times I've needed it (once to remove a deeply embedded splinter, once to make a field repair to my backpack) I was glad to have it along. There's no way to predict when you'll need a sharp blade, right?

5. **FIRE STARTER**: Some people like to carry candle stubs, others carry some sort of chemicals.

Me? I carry an old film canister (which is now a highly coveted vintage item) filled with dryer lint coated with petroleum jelly. I also carry a few tea light candles in case I have to start a fire using damp wood.

Pick what seems most sensible for your hiking terrain, and double wrap it in plastic to keep it dry.

6. **MATCHES**: What good are your knife and fire starter if you can't start a fire?

Don't bring book matches; because they get damp and might not ignite in less-than-ideal conditions. Wooden matches, double bagged in plastic, work well. Spring for the weatherproof kind with large coated heads, and you're guaranteed a flame.

If you want to carry a lighter, just be sure it's in working condition and filled with fuel.

Another dose of common sense: **Fire starter materials**, along with **matches**, are only going to be useful if you have fuel to burn. Desert hiking, rocky alpine terrain, arctic tundra – probably not going to be able to sustain a fire for long there!

If you hike in these types of areas, fall back on extra layers of clothing, along with high fat foods, to maintain body temperature until daylight.

Tip: If your hiking takes you to areas with plentiful dead fall, dried grasses or animal dung to burn, be sure you have the skills to get a fire going. Hypothermia is no joke, plus a fire can keep your spirits up and serve as a beacon for searchers.

7. **FIRST AID KIT**: You can buy a very complete kit, but it's probably a bit much for a dayhike on established trails. You can cobble a very serviceable one together on your own by raiding your bathroom cabinets.

What do you absolutely need in your **dayhike first aid kit**? As with so many other hiking tips, it depends somewhat upon where you are hiking.

For instance, snakebite supplies are not needed on the Pacific Northwest trails west of the Cascade Mountain range, but make sense in Eastern Washington and the desert Southwest.

However, there are some universal essentials no hiker should be without:

-pain relief,

-antiseptic,

-soap or sanitizer,

-band aids,

-gauze,

-cotton balls, and tweezers.

8. **FLASHLIGHT**: A **flashlight** revisits the theme of clear vision on a hiking trail.

Sometimes events unfold to keep you on the trail past sunset, and you'll be faced with a choice of staying put until daybreak (as you deploy some ofthe other items on your essentials list), or hiking through darkness (a navigational challenge).

Either way, a flashlight is going to help you. A waterproof lightweight one using LED illumination is essential on your dayhiking pack list.

A headlamp can be used instead, leaving both hands free to navigate in the dark.

Just remember to do a battery check when you switch out your pack contents at the turn of the season.

And turn the batteries around while storing the illumination device, so there's no chance of triggering an accidental "ON" position in the murky depths of your pack.

9. **TOPOGRAPHIC MAP**: A **map and compass** are useless if you don't know how to use them.

However, a map is less useless than a compass because it can give you at least a vague idea of where you are in relation to the trailhead, nearest road, and water sources.

If you're relying on maps loaded on an electronic device like your cell phone, be mindful of battery life as you check your position. And don't be shocked when cell coverage is less than ideal in dense forests, at the bottom of canyons, or in mountainous area (Chapter 7).

That's why I recommend that you carry paper maps with you, take them out during rest breaks, and study them. It's also a great form of entertainment at your lunch spot: play "name that peak" as you munch your lunch.

And be sure to check out Google Earth and World Wind for fantastic satellite images and well marked maps for any spot you're heading to.

Hiking with a mental map already in place makes everything easier if something disrupts your dayhike.

10. **COMPASS**: Goes along with the map on your hiking pack list, right? But only if you know what to do with the little gizmo. Take a navigational course if compasses confound you.

Your cell phone will help you navigate, but it's only as good as its charge and signal.

Chapter 7 gives you other navigational options to consider.

There you have it: the bare-bones essentials hiking pack list. Ho-hum, right? *Just common sense.*

That's exactly right. **Common sense** can get you through all sorts of scrapes.

Look over the list again. Notice how there are safety and comfort **"themes"** embedded in the list.

For example: If you're lost and are going to stay put for the night, you **need to stay warm** (extra clothes, fire starter, knife and matches) and **not hungry** (extra food and water - a great aid for thinking clearly in an emergency situation).

If you make the decision to travel in search of your original destination or back to the trail head, you need these to **navigate safely**: sunglasses to reduce daylight glare, or a flashlight at night, plus a map and compass.

And if there's an **injury?** You need to deal with it efficiently with your first aid kit, knife, extra food, shelter & warm clothing until help arrives or you can walk out.

Ten Essentials Revisited

Don't be afraid to personalize your ten essentials list. Here are a few trail-tested ideas:

1. **EMERGENCY SHELTER**: A lightweight, waterproof tarp can be converted into shelter using your trekking poles or downed tree limbs.

It can act as an insulating layer on the ground when you break for lunch, or be used to drag wood or an injured trail buddy.

There are thinner "mylar" types of space blankets, but don't expect them to stand up to very much wear and tear. However, their reflective surface could be used to signal help, or to wrap around an injured hiker to conserve body heat.

2. **WATER TREATMENT**: Bringing water treatment technology along is an absolute necessity if you are doing anything other than a straightforward day hike on a popular trail.

You can only go a few days without water, and it might take that long to get rescued.

Locate surface water on your map, and drink it untreated if you have to.

Although you can only last a few days without water, weigh the risk of a possible Giardia infection against the dire consequences of dehydration, and drink up.

3. EMERGENCY REPAIR SUPPLIES: These are versatile, lightweight items that can be pressed into service for repairs of clothing and gear. Think about things you probably already have, such as:

-pliable and tough nylon cord,

-strong safety pins,

-needle and thread,

-rubber bands,

-duct tape,

-nylon cable ties ("zip" ties) of various lengths,

-zip lock bags in several sizes,

-a few extra bootlaces.

Tip: Wind lots of duct tape around your water bottle. Use it for blister prevention, field repairs to equipment, and patching holes in clothing or gear.

4. PEN AND PAPER: If you get into a jam, chances are you will be rattled and confused about what to do.

Have the mental discipline to sit yourself down to write down a description of the last spot you knew where you were. For instance: "I remember passing a moss covered log across the trail not too long ago, where the creek crossed the trail."

Then use your map and time keeping device to figure out:

-Where did you leave the trail, and why?

-How long ago? Can you verify it, or are you guessing?

-Which recent major landmarks can you recall?

If you can't back track for some reason in your physical reality, at least you can get a mental grip and fight off the panicky feeling that always leads to bad decisions. Write out at least one "rescue" scenario, and calculate how much time and effort it might take.

Doing these things will calm you, give you purpose and might lead to more (better?) ideas.

Another use for pen and paper: Leave a note detailing your situation somewhere along the trail for others to find.

I'm sure you can think of other uses for paper, too (such as adding to your hiking pack list on the fly, fire starter, fly swatter...).

Just be sure the paper is weatherproof.

5. **BABY WIPES**: Not just for babies! Be sure these make it onto your hiking pack list for use as toilet paper, or to clean hands prior to eating.

NOTE: Use a dedicated zip lock bag to pack used wipes back home for proper disposal. Hiding it under a rock is not cool because local wildlife or windy conditions can create an unsightly mess. You wouldn't appreciate used toilet paper in your living room, would you?

6. **BANDANNA**: This small square of fabric can become indispensable on the trail. Just a few quick ideas:

-an emergency eye patch,

-a towel to cool your head and neck during a heat wave,

-for unexpected feminine hygiene needs (filled with moss and attached with safety pins, you get the idea),

-a bug swatter,

-two of them tied together as a halter top on an unexpectedly hot day.

7. **INSECT REPELLENT** might also be necessary on your hiking pack list, if only to preserve your sanity long enough to come up with an emergency plan.

ADD THIS TO YOUR LIST: INTUITION

Many, many jokes have been made about female intuition, also called "hunches". So it must be real, right?

And Spiderman's got his "spidey sense", so this inner wisdom is common to both genders.

Seriously, as a hiker it pays to use this inbuilt "uh oh" detector. If you think something looks or feels wrong, don't ignore that information.

Pay attention when you get the tingles, or when a surprising thought flashes across your mind.

The obvious place to use your intuition is when you meet strangers on the trail, especially ones who are dressed inappropriately or are acting very "non-hikerish" (see Chapter 5).

Example: Meeting a spaced out looking person dressed in blue jeans, a tank top and flip flops and no backpack on a cool spring morning, who asks you what time it is with a dazed expression. Hikers don't behave that way!

Another example: Anyone who looks nervous or overly interested in you as you approach. Most hikers are content to mind their own business, and will have limited interest in you.

Realize that you are under no obligation to answer questions, reveal your name or destination, or stand there chit chatting if you feel uncomfortable. Move past anyone who gives you the tingles quickly without letting your inner voice scold you about being rude.

Here's another example of when to tune into your gut.

The weather is turning breezy and colder minute by minute, and it looks like rain clouds moving in. Your trail buddy is oblivious, or hell bent on reaching the destination.

You know that you aren't prepared to spend the night huddled under a tree.

Do you speak up? Or just live with your intuition screeching in the privacy of your own thoughts?

These examples provide ways to stretch your comfort zone regarding safety, just a little bit. If you don't go into avoidance mode or speak up, why not?

Put your safety first, with manners or politeness a distant second.

Because at the end of the day, intuition is just another way of saying "trust your gut check". It's a trail essential every bit as important as extra food and water.

Chapter Two Summed Up

As a hiker, you are assuming responsibility for your own well being.

You could "just wing it" and react to circumstances as they arise, but a better plan is to have a plan for what you're carrying in your pack.

Which means you have to plan what it's your pack, and know how to use it.

This chapter covered all of the reasons you should carry the ten essentials on every hike.

These essentials are designed to keep you safe, comfortable and able to navigate back to the trail head, no matter what may occur during your hike.

Don't rob yourself of these essentials by cutting corners or forgetting to replenish supplies.

You're smarter than that!

Chapter Two Take-Aways

The ten hiking essentials revolve around **common sense and forethought**.

In no particular order, the **ten essentials include** extra food & extra water, extra clothing, sunglasses, knife, fire starter, matches, first aid, flashlight, map and compass.

Carry these essentials of **safety and comfort** on every day hike, regardless of how short or easy you think the hike will be.

Go beyond the list of ten essentials to create your own safety, comfort and peace of mind.

Include **intuition** on your list of essentials.

Chapter Two Resources

Hiking For Her's Essential Recommendations

Let's take this in the order the ten essentials were discussed in this chapter, shall we?

1. **Extra food and water:** See Chapter 3 for details on what to eat and drink on the trail. I opt for metal water bottles on most dayhikes, and try to have a little extra in my Kleen Kanteen or Hydroflask at the end of every hike.

2. **Extra clothing:** See Chapter 1 Resources for the brands and styles I wear.

3. **Sunglasses:** If you'd like to read all about why wearing polarized sunglasses make you a smart hiker, visit the HFH website.

4. **Knife:** Don't think you'll ever need one? Consider these likely scenarios for when a sharp blade is important:

-To do whatever needs doing in a first aid situation.

-To cut open the toe of your boot to allow you to limp back to the trailhead with massive blisters or an injury.

-To prepare some kindling for starting a fire.

-Or to gut a fish for emergency rations.

You just never know when you'll need a sharp edge, as in a small Swiss Army knife. That's what I carry.

5. **Fire starter:** To make sure you can start a fire if you really need one, carry something flammable. Then know how to use it.

6. **Matches:** If you're going to carry a way to start a fire, put together a kit: matches, striker and case! You'll never even feel this important essential in your pack, but you'll love having it if you need it.

Some folks rely upon lighters. Make sure yours is in working order before trusting it enough to include in your Ten Essentials.

7. **First aid supplies:** You can buy a very complete kit. Or you can carry a lightweight, minimalist kit.

It all depends on how accident prone you and your trail buddies are.

I always carry the complete kit, even on dayhikes, but that's just little worrywart me. Or should I say ex-Girl Scout? Be prepared!

8. **Illumination:** I carry a headlamp rather than a flashlight, because it's a good idea to leave both hands free to navigate in the dark.

But a lightweight flashlight, using LED illumination, would be a good idea on your hiking pack list for short dayhikes when the odds are with you in terms of getting back to the trailhead before dark.

9. **Map(s):** Read Chapter 5 for all the details about how maps are essential items.

10. **Compass:** Learn to navigate confidently using the aforementioned map and a compass, and you'll never have to say you're sorry to a search and rescue team.

Ten Essentials Revisited

I think you noticed that I recommend carrying a few other things for safety and comfort on your dayhikes. Let's take a peek at my favorites.

Insect repellents: DEET is a heavy duty approach to keeping biting insects at bay. I carry full strength when I'm in Alaska and other notoriously buggy environments. Zika, West Nile, and other viruses can't get into your body if mosquitoes don't land on your skin, right?

To avoid toxicities, you might be interested in natural insect repellents. I've had good (but not complete) success with herbal brands in buggy terrain. It smells better than DEET, that's for sure.

Ever seen your arms, legs, torso, and face covered *simultaneously* with mosquitoes eager to drain you dry? You need a light weight bug net.

Emergency shelter: I do carry one of the lightweight thin sheets of mylar in my pack, to be used as a reflective surface to signal my location from the air. But I find that it's too thin to stand up to much wind or rain.

That's why I am never without my trusty tarp.

Sunscreen: It just makes sense to block UV rays from damaging your skin on a day hike.

Neutrogena is the brand my dermatologist recommends, and what I use routinely year round.

I buy several small tubes and put them in my car and my backpacks. That way I'm never caught out in the sun without protection. Combined with my recommended sun hats (Chapter 1 Resources), you'll be well protected.

Reapplying sunscreen every 2 hours is recommended. But how many of us do that while we're enjoying Mother Nature's beauty?

Make it a priority if you're light skinned and/or have a family history of skin cancer.

Waterproof paper: You want the kind that is *guaranteed* weatherproof. And to be extra sure, keep it in a plastic bag.

Baby wipes: Wipes are more durable than toilet paper, and can provide a solution to getting your hands clean before you eat. Be sure your baby wipes are unscented. Why attract more attention from insects?

Seat cushion: Something soft and cushy to sit on. I love cold wet rocks just as much as the next hiker, but sometimes I love a warm, dry caboose better. Thermarest makes abbreviated pads for just this purpose.

A **small, fast drying towel** is indispensable for drying off feet after a stream crossing, or for wiping sweat off your neck (or get it wet and drape it on your hot neck).

And a few more ideas:

*A metal bowl or cup with a handle to melt snow or boil river water, hold berries, or catch rain water.

*A sturdy unbreakable whistle or other low tech **signaling device** such as a lightweight unbreakable signal mirror, or an old CD.

*An illustrated, laminated **list of wild edibles** in your area (in case you can't remember and don't want to risk being poisoned on top of everything else in an emergency situation).

Hiking For Her's Additional Information on Hiking Ten Essentials

Use any of the Ten Essential words to search for more information on the Hiking For Her website.

A few more ideas from the website to keep you safe on the trail:

How To Use A Hiking Journal

Survival Kit

Dealing With Trail Stress

Visit the American Hiking Society for more information on what's essential for hikers to carry.

The United States Geologic Survey (USGS) website has a wealth of information on topographic maps. Look for their FAQs, as well as an article on How To Use A Compass.

Chapter 3: Trail Nutrition

What you eat translates directly into how you think, feel and perform on the trail.

This chapter is all about choosing the right food to keep you full of energy and at your mental best during your hike.

In Chapter 3 you will learn:

-The importance of The Big Three nutrients: carbohydrates, protein, fats

-How to maintain your energy level on a dayhike

-Why water is a vital nutrient for hikers

-The best trail snacks for portability, nutrient density, taste, and digestibility

-Your best dayhike lunch options

-Why hiking chocolate is good news for day hikers

TRAIL NUTRITION

Hiking nutrition may not be the *first* thing you consider when planning a day hike. But it should be!

The reality: Your body needs fuel before, during, **and** after your hike.

If you use a vehicle analogy, it makes lots of sense: in your car, gasoline is fuel while in your body, fuel is calories from food. Both forms of fuel are burned (oxidized), and produce not only energy but waste products such as heat, carbon dioxide and water.

So as you read this chapter, consider your body as your hiking vehicle, requiring proper fuel to get you where you're going on the trail. But it's going to take a few "fill ups" along the way.

Here's one more vehicle analogy before we jump into the details.

Your brain is programmed to send strong signals of hunger when you're running low on fuel in your bloodstream. Hunger pangs are like the "empty" indicator of a car's fuel gauge.

So that explains the big appetite that goes along with big hikes!

Tip: This big calorie burn can be used to your advantage if you're hiking for weight loss.

Big 3 Nutrients Demystified

Let's start with these one-liners to help you remember each of the 3 major nutrient groups:

Carbohydrates conquer the trail with **sustained energy**.

Protein provides **power** via strong muscles.

Fats fill you up and satisfy (satiate) you.

The secret to good trail performance lies in the ratio of these nutrients.

Time for a close look at each of them.

Carbohydrates: Ideal Dayhike Food

Carbohydrates are the most important nutrient to include in your dayhike lunch sack, because they provide fast fuel to your cells.

Carbohydrates are just a fancy way of saying *sugars,* either "*simple*" or "*complex*". Simple is best for quick bursts of energy, but complex wins the day for sustained energy release.

Why is that?

Simple sugars will flood your cell receptors with glucose ("Whoa! Burst of energy!"), then leave you to crash and burn ("Outta gas, I gotta sit down"). It's literally a feast, then famine, scenario in your bloodstream.

Candy bars, sugar coated energy bars, and sugary drinks are notorious for that quick hit of energy, but you should avoid relying on them for sustained energy on the trail. That's when you turn to complex carbohydrates.

But before we leave "the simples" behind, let's note that they do have their place in your dayhike routine.

Example: Before conquering a long steep trail section, consume a candy bar with lots of nuts. Nuts act as a source of fat/protein and fiber to slow down the release of the sugar. They provide a more sustained, even release of nutrients so you can tackle the trail.

Tip: Snickers are favorite dayhike food for thru hikers (yes, it's spelled that way), those dedicated hikers who specialize in serial day hikes for weeks and months at a time.

Of course, a chocolate coated candy bar presents other issues for a dayhiker:

-Will it melt and leak into your ten essentials? (Chapter 2)

-Is it packaged in layers of wrapping that you have to keep track of? (Leave No Trace, Chapter 7)

-Will it crumble to dust at the bottom of your pack?

-Will it give you indigestion if you wolf it down while hiking?

-Will it make you crave water (Hydration, Chapter 4), thus depleting your water supply? (Ten Essentials, Chapter 2)

-Can your pancreas (and mood) handle the sudden rise in blood sugar, followed by the crash?

See? Those simple sugars called candy bars are not so simple after all!

Maybe a different trail snack is a better choice (coming right up).

Here's a different way to incorporate simple sugars into your dayhike: Suck on hard candy when you have to work hard on steep uphill sections of the trail.

If your day pack has a crafty little zippered pocket (see Chapter 1) within easy reach on the hip belt or shoulder strap, stash your favorite candy there. These little flavor bombs keep your mouth hydrated (the saliva reflex), and take your mind off the hard work at hand (straight up bribery).

And because the sugar is released quickly and steadily, skeletal muscles are constantly fueled and satisfied brain cells keep you alert. Such a deal from a little piece of sweetness!

Heads up: If you're sensitive to, or politically opposed to, high fructose corn syrup, be careful about buying cheap bags of candy because the cheaper it is, the more likely it is to contain the stuff.

Read the labels! In fact, read all of the labels on the ingredients that go into your trail food.

Avoid preservatives, excessive amounts of sugar (which can masquerade under many names including glucose, fructose, sucrose, corn syrup, and many more), flavoring chemicals and artificial coloring. These make your organs of elimination, especially your liver, work overtime while adding little to the nutritional bottom line.

Tip: If you know you're allergic to an ingredient, you might not see it listed on the label, because in the U.S. the label can use vague terms such as "flavoring". Visit the product's website, or call customer support, to be really sure.

Don't try out a new food on the trail if you have food sensitivities, because you don't want to trigger a reaction when you're away from help.

If you need to carry an "epi pen" filled with epinephrine to reverse an allergic reaction, be sure your trail buddies know where you store it in your pack, and how to use it.

To sum up the carbohydrate story thus far:

Simple carbohydrates yield quick, fleeting bursts of energy.

Sustained Energy: Complex Carbohydrates

Throughout most of the day on the trail, your goal is slow and sustained energy release.

That's where **complex carbohydrates** from grains or fruit, coupled with a dash of protein, come into the picture - and your lunch sack - as appropriate dayhike foods.

If you'd like details on how to calculate your exact nutrition needs as a dayhiker, I recommend my e-booklet on this very subject, which you can pick up by visiting the Amazon page where you purchased this book. I created it based on the questions lots of dayhikers were asking about what to eat on the trail.

If you're serious about good trail performance as a dayhiker, the information in this inexpensive, instant download booklet will get you pointed in the right direction (so to speak). There's also one for gluten free hiking, if you need to go GF on the trail.

But for now, let's just go with the handy little rule that says "40% of your trail food" should be devoted to carbohydrates.

How often to snack?

Here's the pivotal question: How often to stop and snack?

Some dayhikers like to stop every hour to snack on handfuls of trail mix or gorp, or to gulp down an energy bar (see Chapter 3 Resources for recommendations).

Unfortunately, stopping often to eat may work against you. As your body tries to digest the frequent food, blood is being diverted from legs and arms to your gastrointestinal tract. You'll feel sluggish and your pace will drop.

It's also hard to get into a good trail rhythm if you're stopping a lot to unwrap treats or chase a snack with water.

For these reasons, I prefer to rely on my stored glycogen and fat for the first few hours of a day hike, then stop for a snack when I receive strong hunger signals. (This depends upon what I had for breakfast, the type of terrain, and the temperature, too.)

That gnawing sensation after a few hours forces me to stop and break out a handful of trail mix or an energy bar, along with plenty of water to wash it all down.

The water isn't just a way of getting the peanut butter off the roof of my mouth. Nope, it's a ***cellular energy insurance policy***!

Water is a solvent, and if you don't have enough of it in your body, your nutrients won't be broken down and absorbed. As a result, your energy levels will suffer (see section on hiking water below, as well as Hydration, Chapter 4).

Protein and Fats

Long story short: Don't skip these! But don't overindulge, either.

Here's a glimpse of the little protein dance your body does every day:

Protein provides building blocks for strong muscles, active enzymes to break down food, and stable cell membranes, plus many other parts of normal body function (physiology).

As you hike, you use your skeletal muscles hard, and they have to be fueled with carbohydrates constantly to keep you going strong. But protein keeps those muscles strong.

That means protein needs to be part of your hiking lunch, as well as your daily diet.

Where you decide to get your protein is up to you: animals or plants. But skipping protein on a dayhike is a mistake.

Fats have gotten a scary bad name in the media, but the fact remains that without high quality fat molecules your body can't build strong cell membranes, send electrical messages efficiently, or store fuel for periods of low calorie intake.

But there's an even more important reason to eat fat on a day hike: **satiety**. That means you'll feel satisfied after eating lunch. You don't want to fight hunger pangs and that empty feeling when you want to concentrate on the trail, right?

While 40% of your day hike calories should come from carbohydrates, protein and fat should each make up 30%. That gets us to 100%, right?

No need to be exact about these proportions on a day hike, just a general rule to keep in mind. Reading food labels will clue you into the approximate amounts of hiking nutrients that your trail snacks and lunch provide.

But you can use your own body cues on the trail, too.

If you don't feel full after lunch, you might need more a bit more fat on your sandwich: a slice of cheese, a spoonful of nut butter, or half of an avocado.

Or try coconut cookies or oily fish as lunch options.

If you feel sluggish just an hour into your hike, add more carbs to your snack bag next time. And tweak your breakfast: did you eat enough complex carbs such as oatmeal before hitting the trail?

Here's my personal favorite: Legs feel like cement? No desire to power your pack up a hill? Snack on jerky or nuts for a protein boost.

Heads up: If you consume *too much protein and/or fat* in your hiking snacks and lunch, you'll feel sluggish while your digestive system works hard to process them.

Fats pass through the stomach without much digestive activity, but protein needs a lot of stomach acid (and time) to be broken down. You don't want to load yourself up only to slow yourself down, do you?

Protein and fat also takes more water in the digestive tract to process them, so you'll have to drink more. This translates into a heavier pack, or stopping to purify surface water to fill up your water bottle.

Bottom line for protein and fats: carry tasty, easy to digest options and be sure to monitor your energy level and stamina in case you're not eating enough of them.

HOW TO MAINTAIN YOUR ENERGY LEVEL

The human body has a remarkable capacity for handling hourly fluctuations in fuel.

If your car has an empty fuel tank, it shuts down. But if **you** have an empty fuel tank (your stomach & blood vessels), all of your systems remain online, at least for a while. Why is that?

Your hard working liver, and to a limited extent your skeletal muscles, deliver a steady supply of "fuel" to your cells in the form of glucose (the sugar molecule preferred by most cells, already mentioned above). This is a universal "cell rule", whether or not you're hiking.

Thus, a steady blood glucose level (the key to maintaining energy level) is the responsibility of your liver as you hike. But your liver needs your help.

If you've eaten a decent breakfast, and plan to stop for a snack after a reasonable interval of hiking, your liver has no trouble delivering a steady stream of fuel (glucose) to your contracting skeletal muscles, your brain, your heart, and all other parts of your body: in other words, maintaining energy level to meet demand.

Sugars from your breakfast carbohydrates will be available in the bloodstream until lunch time, thanks to your dependable and multitasking liver.

The liver also depends upon stored sugar (glycogen), which it saved from excess sugar in previous meals. Did you eat pasta, starchy grains, vegetables and bread the day before your hike? Good job! That's how glycogen gets stashed away for later use on the trail.

Note the word "decent" tied to "meal". A sugary doughnut and a cup of coffee as you drive to the trail head? Sure, that will work as trail food, but you're forcing your body to work harder than it should to regulate your blood sugar within fairly tight limits over long spans of time.

Yo-yo spikes of blood sugar are harmful in the long run, because they stress out the pancreas (an accessory organ of digestion) and will impede its ability to supply a hormone called insulin.

Without insulin, the sugar in your blood can't get into your cells: The cells begin to drown in an ocean of sugar, calling out for sugar, thirsting for sugar....but not being able to take it in and use it for fuel.

Eventually, major organ systems begin to lose function: eyes, kidneys, immune system... that's called diabetes, and it's a chronic, life altering condition that no hiker wants to deal with.

Instead of doughnuts and coffee, how about a bowl of oatmeal with a spoonful of brown sugar or maple syrup, plus a handful of walnuts and dried fruit?

Or fill your breakfast bowl with a hearty grain such as quinoa, topped with fruit and almond milk.

That type of breakfast provides "slow burn" fuel to keep you going until your first snack break. Glucose is released from the food into your bloodstream over several hours rather than in a burst right after you eat.

Bonus: Your liver doesn't have to scramble to regulate the amount of sugar entering your bloodstream by cutting up stored glycogen molecules into glucose.

Now you know how to avoid long term trouble with energy fluctuations on the trail: avoid large doses of sugary nutrient-poor foods and opt for whole (unprocessed, unrefined, unadulterated) foods.

Tips for maintaining energy level on your hike

*Make time for breakfast, even if that means getting up a half hour earlier. If you're one of those people who pride themselves on "never eating breakfast", try seeing this choice through the eyes of your hard working pancreas and liver.

*If the thought of eating breakfast makes you nauseous, how about sipping a smoothie on the way to the trailhead? You can make it the night before, and give it a good shake before consuming it. Whether you call it a shake or a smoothie is up to you!

*When you get strong hunger signals on the trail, stop within a few minutes for a snack. Frequent, small amounts of easily digested food are easier on your digestive system than one big intake of fatty or protein rich foods. Waiting too long forces the brain to get more insistent: headache, dizziness, nausea.

*Carry a small bag of trail mix in a shirt pocket or accessible pack pocket, and munch while you hike. Don't overdo this, because you want your blood flowing to your legs rather than to your digestive system.

*Snack on raw nuts and seeds mixed with unsulfured, unsweetened dried fruits (the ones that look kind of sketchy and shriveled). Chew them slowly and thoughtfully to grind them into small enough pieces for optimal digestion and absorption.

*Hydration is the key to absorbing your nutrients. Water breaks, or frequent sips from your hydration bladder, are essential to maintaining energy.

*If you are planning lots of elevation gain and lots of distance during your hike, your body will ask for a slow steady release of energy throughout the day. Use the 40-30-30 rule to plan your dayhike food, with plenty of time to sit and enjoy your snacks and your lunch.

*If you're facing a flat, slow hike, you can get away with less food planning and make up your calorie deficit with a hearty dinner.

*Underlying all of this nutrient intake is how well you digest your food. Just because you chew and swallow it doesn't mean you absorb and utilize it.

Eating small snacks more frequently might be easier on the digestive system, which needs to keep supplying glucose and other nutrients such as calcium to the skeletal muscles as they contract and relax.

If you experience digestive upsets such as burping, indigestion or altered bowel movements, figure out which food is making you upset. This might take a little detective work, so keep notes on what you ate when you felt bad and compare it with hikes when you felt great.

*Thoughtful chewing also leads to better nutrient digestion, beginning with your salivary amylase (a carbohydrate enzyme in your mouth) and providing more surface area for stomach and intestinal enzymes to break apart large food molecules.

I know, TMI (too much information).

*In the middle of a hike is NOT the best place to try new foods, or new flavors of old favorites. I have done this, and regretted it every time.

Being hungry due to unpalatable (or downright inedible) food robs you of hiking enjoyment. But more importantly, it deprives you of much needed nutrients for your hard working body when you toss uneaten food back into your lunch sack.

These tips give you multiple ways to maintain your energy levels during your hike. Try at least one, and be amazed at how much further you can go, and feel great doing it!

HIKING WATER: AN IMPORTANT NUTRIENT

This may seem odd to you, but water is a required daily nutrient in your diet, every bit as important as carbohydrates, proteins and fats.

That's why you have thirst programmed into your brain as a basic drive.

Without adequate water in your bloodstream and tissues, it's harder for your body to eliminate waste, utilize oxygen, manufacture important biomolecules for energy production, or repair damaged structures such as micro-tears in your muscles.

The right type of water, at the right time and in the right amount, is essential to feeling good on the trail. That's why staying hydrated should be a top priority on any trail.

Tip: Never ignore thirst signals. Do whatever it takes to get water into your system, because by the time your brain relays a strong desire for water to your conscious mind, you're already dehydrated to some degree.

Lack of water works against you by rewarding your stubbornness ("I don't want to stop for water right now") with muscle cramps, confused thinking, and worse.

What about water in the form of sports drinks? That's a personal decision, but there are two things to consider:

Do you need to consume extra sugars along with artificial colors and preservatives (and pay a premium price for them)?

And do you really need a liquid dose of electrolytes (salts such as potassium and sodium) to combat the depleting effects of sweating?

If you're hiking in triple digit heat, maybe the answer is yes. But for a moderate length hike in moderate weather, maybe not.

Chapter 4 is all about hiking water, so check there for answers to your hydration questions.

BEST TRAIL SNACKS

Trail snacks: as if hiking itself isn't reason enough to put your boots on!

These yummy mouthfuls of snacking goodness don't have to be expensive or complicated, unless you want them to be.

You can make it your mission to cruise the aisles of any grocery store and find plenty of companies who want you to try their latest & greatest snacks.

But be careful!

You want food that works with you, not against you, on your hikes.

So avoiding preservatives, additives, processed sugar, fillers, and weird or salty flavorings is definitely in your best interest as a hiker.

Skip the snacks made of long lists of words you can't pronounce. In fact, the shorter the ingredient list, the better if you look at it from a cellular perspective.

On a day hike, the weight of your food probably isn't a worry unless you have a knee or back injury that you need to be mindful of -OR- you will be carrying other gear such as a heavy camera lens, tripod, field guides, or a water filter.

And the less packaging around your food, the better. You won't drop any plastic wrappers on the trail, you don't have to keep track of them in a stiff breeze, and there's less to cart home as trash.

It's also cheaper to buy in bulk, and repackage the food into dayhike appropriate portions. And you can feel good about your smaller environmental footprint.

How to pick great trail snacks

You definitely want to carry and consume snacks that sustain a steady blood glucose level (no "crash and burn", as outlined above).

AND you want snacks that are compact, lightweight, yet nutrient dense. Throw in tasty, just for fun.

Are there any trail snacks on the planet that deliver all of that??

Actually, yes. Read on for a glimpse into the wonderful world of Hiking For Her approved best trail snacks.

Favorite Dayhike Foods: Trail Bars

Not the "cocktails" kind of bars! I'm referring to those you make at home, or trail bars you buy to keep you going between meals during a hike.

To be on the sanctioned HFH list, trail bars have got to be delicious, nutritious AND they must pass focused scrutiny of their ingredients.

Chapter 3 Resources will name names on tried and true trail snacks.

Another thing to look for is the ability to buy these snacks in bulk. If you purchase them one at a time, the price adds up fast.

So if you can get a good deal on a case of trail bars, toss some into the freezer and use up the rest in a short amount of time (a month or so; check expiration dates).

They are great for snacks at work or while commuting, too. Stash a few in your car, purse and desk drawer.

Even better: if your kids will eat them after soccer practice!

If you want to go organic with your trail food, there are tips on the HFH website.

NOTE: Be sure to purchase high quality nuts if you make your own trail bars and snack mixes. If nuts have been sitting around at room temperature for awhile, the fats become rancid.

Avoid rancid nuts at all costs (meaning high quality nuts will cost more but be worth it). Pass up bargain priced nuts that sit in bulk bins exposed to light and air for a long time. They might be cheaper in price, but will definitely deliver sub-par nutrients.

Sometimes you'll notice the "off" flavor of rancidity, but not always if there are strong competing flavors.

Tip: Keep your nuts in the freezer to preserve their oils, especially when you can't get out on the trail as often as you'd like.

Some hikers need to be gluten free. More and more people are choosing (or needing) to avoid gluten, and the marketplace is happy to provide GF options for the trail. See Chapter 3 Resources for the bars I rely on (GF for over 2 decades, and counting).

Tip: If you're experiencing bloating, gas and general digestive unease after you eat, play around with gluten free food to see if it brings you some relief.

BEST DAYHIKE LUNCHES

When you finally stop on the trail for lunch, you want easy to eat food with complex carbohydrates predominating, along with protein and fat. Recall that the ratio of these nutrients should be 40C/30P/30F.

Dayhike sandwich suggestions on the bread, bagel, tortilla or crackers of your choice:

-peanut butter and sliced banana,

-almond butter and fruit spread,

-tofu "egg salad" - extra spicy! with lettuce,

-curried chicken salad with lots of crunchy celery and cashews,

-cheese, turkey slices, spicy greens & mustard,

-tuna & avocado.

Notice that each combo has protein and fat, paired with the healthy doses of carbohydrates you need for sustained energy.

Another great source of protein is jerky (dried meat). But beware! Not all jerky is created equal.

Some jerkies (as most jerks) aren't good for you. They are chock full of preservatives, salt, and strong flavorings that deaden your taste buds and make you crave water.

Instead, buy jerky that boasts minimal processing, lack of nitrites and nitrates, and freshness. All of this information is available on the label.

Live it up a little, and branch out from beef jerky to try pork, salmon, bison, and lamb. (My apologies to the vegans among us. Soy jerky can be a trusted protein source on the trail.)

Tip: Try bison/buffalo jerky because it seems to "burn clean", an important consideration for day hike foods. Burns clean translates into no digestive upsets and no nasty flavor burps.

Tip: Buy a small package of an exotic jerky (salmon, venison, goat) before committing to an expensive large pouch. Some of these are an acquired taste.

A few more tips for dayhike lunches:

*If you're used to racing through lunch, dial into your surroundings and mindfully consume your sandwich with slow, thoughtful chewing. Let lunch nourish you on more than one level.

*Did you know that the *American food supply* contains over 3000 ingredients to boost flavor, extend shelf life, and create certain textures? That's a lot of chemicals!!

Strive to avoid preservatives and artificial ingredients which keep your liver & kidneys distracted from their important tasks: pulling nutrients from your bloodstream and dumping waste products via urine and feces.

*Be careful with strong artificial flavors. You don't want your taste buds to become jaded by fake flavorings, lots of salt and sugar, or intense flavor combinations. Why miss out on savoring the subtle flavors in great dayhike foods?

Plus, these strong flavors make you crave water, which might be a limited commodity in your pack.

*Sometimes paying more for the convenience of prepared trail food is worth it. Calculate the value of your time and decide if you'd rather put your attention on planning the hiking destination (Chapter 5), not the menu.

HIKING CHOCOLATE

Hiking chocolate: it's not just for breakfast any more!

No, really, chocolate deserves a place on a hiker's list of go-to foods, for plenty of sound scientific reasons.

And let's just be honest: it tastes great!

Maybe you've read about the latest research highlighting its heart-protective benefits, or heard a news blurb about chocolate as a *wonder food*. Chocolate is the new kale.

But I believe a few ***words of caution*** are in order. Not every type of chocolate is the "good" kind for hikers, even if it *tastes* good.

So let's take a look at why hiking chocolate is good for you, and then throw in a few cautions.

The first thing to consider when selecting hiking chocolate is the amount of **antioxidants** the chocolate contains.

Anti what?? Aren't we pro-chocolate?

Well, to keep it short and sweet, as a hiker you need to consume molecular oxygen in order to make energy at the cellular level (adenosine triphosphate in our mitochondria, to be not so short).

The two atoms of oxygen bonded into each atmospheric oxygen molecule can cause trouble in the process, trying to rip off electrons (high energy particles) from nearby molecules.

An anti-oxidant works to protect your cells from these "rogue" destructive oxygen free radicals.

So consuming antioxidants in your diet is a good daily habit, cellularly speaking. For example, arteries are protected against cholesterol oxidation and plaque formation by antioxidants.

And doesn't it make sense for hikers, who are breathing deeply hour after hour on the trail, pulling lots of oxygen molecules through their respiratory system and circulating it via blood vessels through the heart and out to the tissues, to **consume antioxidants**?

You bet it does! So leave room in your lunch bag for some chocolate.

What kind of hiking chocolate is best?

It turns out that **dark chocolate** has lots of flavonoids (plant based antioxidants), with flavanol being the specific type found in cocoa.

Mother Nature puts flavanols into other foods, too: cranberries, onions, red wine, apples. Chocolate + red wine... oops, my mind is wandering off topic here.

It's important to be *discriminating* about the type of chocolate you put into your lunch sack: you want to buy cocoa with high amounts of flavanol. This molecule can be stripped away during processing, and you don't want to waste calories on chocolate that's not protecting your cardiovascular system.

Tip: Look for high percentages of dark chocolate on the label, 70% at the minimum. The higher the percentage, the less sweet your treat. Work your way up to the highest numbers gradually if you're weaning yourself off sweet milk chocolate.

Sadly, what passes for chocolate on American store shelves has been highly processed. Our taste buds have been trained to want sweetened candy bars, which means highly processed white sugar predominates over flavanol.

For example, "Dutch" chocolate has been alkalized - there's not much flavanol left in it. Then it's sweetened. So check the label for the source of cacao, and whether it has been processed.

To complicate this picture, there are lots of low quality fats added to highly processed chocolate. This adds calories, but not necessarily nutrients. It's part of why chocolate has gotten a bad reputation in the hiking nutrition world.

Can you see how what ends up being labeled "chocolate" isn't always that great for a hiker's body?

To be fair, high quality cocoa (cacao) crammed full of flavanols is slightly bitter, and not very palatable by itself. So a sweetener and fat must be added or people won't buy it.

Just watch out for how *MUCH* fat is added.

We've been told that fat is bad for us. Earlier in this chapter we saw how the right fats are an important part of a hiker's diet.

Here's where chocolate is a winner: the cocoa butter used in making *high quality* chocolate has components in it which can either protect (oleic acid) or remain neutral (stearic acid) in terms of your cardiovascular health.

There's more to it than this, but for now, are you with me on the merits of hiking chocolate?

Consume wisely!

Now you know why chocolate is *not* the big, bad food it was once made out to be. It has a legitimate place in your hiking lunch sack.

However, this is not a license to ingest massive amounts of chocolate during a hike. Sorry to put the brakes on such a sweet story.

An ounce here, an ounce there, is a hiker's best approach. Overindulging in chocolate racks up fat calories and plays havoc with your blood sugar levels, things to avoid if you want to keep hiking into your nineties!

So please play around with the source of your chocolate. Don't settle for the icky-sweet, over processed stuff on a random supermarket shelf.

Ferret out the best dark chocolate brands: 55% cacao and higher, with just enough sugar and fat to make them delicious.

In fact, consider this a homework assignment from me. Your task is to locate the best sources for hiking chocolate, do some taste tests (now there's a sweet homework assignment!) and consume it regularly on the trail in small quantities.

Extra credit: sharing it with your trail buddies.

Your new hiking motto

If you're a chocolate lover, or are willing to experiment, don't forego this treat on a hike. Just be smart about it!

Ready?

Repeat after me: *A bit(e) of chocolate makes any trail sweeter!*

Chapter 3 Summed Up

It's a mistake to worry about your gear, your footwear, and your destination without putting some thought into the food you're eating on the trail.

Consider this chapter your call to action.

Not only should you search out the best hiking chocolate as a trail treat, but you can give yourself permission to sample different combinations of carbohydrates, proteins and fats until you have a "greatest hits" list.

You won't regret this investment of time, because you will stay in love with the hiking life all day long. Stamina, endurance, strength, mental clarity, balanced mood – all thanks to your trail food.

Don't forget that one of the Ten Essentials (Chapter 2) is to pack a little *extra food and water*, even for short dayhikes.

If you don't need it on the trail, you have a delicious snack for the ride home.

Chapter 3 Take-Aways

Simple carbohydrates provide quick bursts of energy so consume them at particular times during your hike.

Complex carbohydrates provide the sustained energy you need to tackle a day hike. Eat these at breakfast and lunch.

Proteins and fats support the slow release of fuel into your bloodstream and keep your body feeling **strong and satisfied**. Don't skip these!

The best day hike lunches have balanced nutrients: **40% carbs, 30% protein, 30% fat.**

Snack frequently, but don't overdo it.

Water is an important hiking nutrient so **drink often throughout the hike**, even if you're not thirsty.

Dark chocolate made with high quality cocoa butter, consumed in moderation, deserves a place in your trail snacking repertoire.

Chapter Three Resources

Hiking For Her Recommendations For Trail Food

TRAIL MIX

My best trail tip is to snack on raw nuts and dried fruits, especially if you haven't found an energy bar you really like.

My favorite source for these? Trader Joes.

I absolutely love their Omega Trek Mix or the Go Raw Trek Mix.

But rest assured, you can find lots of other combos.

These handy packs can be easily repackaged into trail sized bags.

Just go easy on them during your hike. A handful, chewed thoughtfully as you check the map for your next benchmark, will do the trick.

If you're a do-it-yourselfer, you already know how to cruise the bulk bins aisles of a grocery store. Just don't let yourself fall into taste ruts (no trail comparisons will be made here).

*Try dried wasabi peas, spicy pecans, candied ginger, chili infused chocolate chunks.

TRAIL BARS

Let's take a glance at the reasons these are my current favorite trail snacks, specifically trail bars (sometimes called energy bars).

1.Lara Bars have been around for awhile. When they first came out, I was overjoyed by how short the ingredient list was - and how much flavor they packed.

These bars rely upon nuts, so if you're nut intolerant (I will skip the easy joke here, and you're welcome) these are not for you.

The variety of flavors is mind boggling. My current favorite is Cashew Cookie, but I have been known to buy a case of mixed flavors to keep my taste buds from dozing off: a variety pack will come to the rescue every time!

2. ZING bars are designed by nutritionists who paid attention to nutrient ratios but also got the taste right.

These bars don't get rock hard in your pack overnight, and they don't melt in the heat (the same could be said of Lara Bars - but Laras will get smooshed if you subject them to high pressures like sitting on your pack).

I love the Zing blueberry flavor, but truthfully, I have yet to meet one I don't like! The chocolate coconut bar really hits the spot sometimes but for some reason I keep gravitating back to blueberry.

These can be quite expensive if purchased one at a time, so consider the bulk buy option and split some with trail buddies.

3. KIND bars are a bit on the sweet side, but if I need lots of glucose in my bloodstream to tackle some serious elevation gain or distance, I enjoy these.

If you like savory and sweet combined, you should try these for sure.

Warning: They rely heavily upon nuts. If you are allergic to a particular type, read the labels. Most of the names shout it right out, such as my current favorite, Almond & Coconut.

Again, variety is the spice of hiking life, so invest in a variety pack if these become your favorite trail snacks.

4. My apologies for the name of this favorite: **Caveman Bars.** This is, after all, a *woman's* hiking book!

However, I'm willing to overlook the name and focus on their taste. Why?

Because I was introduced to these bars on a back country trip through ANWR (Arctic National Wildlife Refuge in Alaska), and they kept me fueled through 10 days of rugged terrain and temperature extremes. I kept looking forward to rest breaks so I could eat another one!

Remember my calorie rule: Calories don't count when you're working hard, so don't count them!

Favorite flavor? I couldn't decide! If Costco is in your area, look for a variety pack there.

5. **Fruit Source:** Do you crave fruity goodness during a hike? Me, too!

Rather than carry a container of raspberries, get a sack of Fruit Source mini bites and divide them into smaller portions.

Their chewiness will take your mind off the mud holes and mosquitoes, too.

6. Interested in making your own "energy spheres" ? Visit the HFH website for the recipe.

Spheres are fast, easy, and totally delicious. And even better:

-You control the quality of the ingredients.

-They are so good for you: natural sources of sugar, high in fiber, and a nice balance of fat, protein, and carbohydrates for slow, sustained energy.

-And did I mention how easily they ride along in your pack?

Warning: spheres convert to discs when sat upon. Consider yourself warned.

JERKY

I found a particularly flavorful and "clean" buffalo jerky because of a stranger's trail recommendation (Yes, I've been known to stop total strangers and ask about something, and this time it was along the lines of "Hmm, what's that? It looks good!").

It's called Tanka Bites, and resembles pemmican in that it combines meat and dried cranberries.

A bit pricey, yes, but geez it's great as trail fuel! So to save some cash while supporting your hard working body, buying in bulk is the only way to go here.

Warning: Pace yourself because you're going to want to gobble it down. The cranberries add a moist deliciousness that is amazing to experience.

Thankfully, this package lasts for several hikes.

And you have my permission to keep this snack all to yourself!

CHOCOLATE

To get you started in your search for hiking chocolate, let me share my favorites with you.

Luckily for me, I live in a city (Seattle, WA, USA) that takes its chocolate VERY seriously, so I have plenty of options for experimenting with a nice balance between nutrition, price, and taste.

My favorite small act of kindness to myself each hiking season is to purchase a new type of hiking chocolate to share on the trail.

In that spirit of sharing trail chocolate (virtually, unfortunately, but you can order some for yourself), here are some of my favorite brands of hiking chocolate.

1. **Theo's Chocolate**. USDA certified organic, fair trade, not cheap but pretty close to heaven.

Currently, my favorite hiking chocolate is the cherry and almond 70% cacao dark chocolate bar.

I find just a small square deeply satisfying. And by buying in bulk and keeping my stash in the freezer, the "per bar" price is much more reasonable than if I buy them one at a time at the grocery store.

Theo's deserves a place in anyone's search for high quality hiking chocolate. You're worth it, don't you think?

And here's another way to pamper yourself: on cool weather hikes, carry a thermos filled to the brim with hot chocolate!

Slide the full thermos into an extra hiking sock, then into the middle of your pack to stay warm. So decadent! And impressive to your trail buddies.

If you prefer peanuts, this one is going to make you smile: Theo's dark chocolate peanut butter cups.

2. **Divine Chocolate.** This company amazes me because it's doing lots of things right: it's 45% owned by the cacao growers, it publishes its annual reports on its website, it cares about its ingredients... AND the chocolate rocks!

Try all of the types until you hit upon your favorite hiking chocolate. Need a hint? Here's my favorite: Divine 70% dark chocolate with raspberries.

3. **Trader Joe's.** Who wouldn't love something named Pound Plus Bittersweet Chocolate?

They deliver a lot of hiking chocolate for not a lot of money, and it's tasty, too.

I like the "with almonds" version. Break it into hunks and throw it into a small zip lock bag. It travels well, and a small amount satisfies as an after lunch snack.

Tip: Fight with your trail buddies over the left overs on the drive home. If there are any!

If you're lucky enough to have access to this store, please check out this chocolate. Or save time - buy it on line!

4. **Newman's Own**: Chocolate-y goodness wrapped around peanut butter. Need I say more?

Rumor has it there's a raspberry version as well.

But what's not to love about peanut butter cups?? I nominate them for the Universal Hiker Trail Food award.

And note their high percentage of heart protective cacao.

HARD CANDIES FOR THE TRAIL

Here are two of my favorite trail hard candies.

The first one tastes like coffee with a hint of caramel cream in it: Werther's Original caramel coffee hard candies.

The original caramel without coffee version is great, too: buttery and very satisfying.

The second option fills your mouth with fruity (organic) goodness, so stock up and stash some in each of your packs!

The variety of flavors is a fun taste treat on the trail, too: Torie & Howard organic hard candies.

Tip: Either of these choices will get stale if left in your pack for too long. Bring only what you'll need for the dayhike, or risk less than ideal textures and flavors.

ELECTROLYTES

Read the next chapter (Chapter 4) for specific information about electrolytes.

For now, here are some recommendations:

I add Ultima powdered electrolytes to my hiking water year round (warmed up in cold weather months; see thermos trick above in Hiking Chocolate).

I'm a fan of the lemon flavor, but all of them taste good.

The other brand I rely upon is NUUN Natural Hydration. You can go a little wild with all of the flavor options, so try them all.

If you're lucky, you'll like every flavor. These give a welcome taste "hit" on a long hike every time you take a sip of your hiking water.

And if your body doesn't need every last little electrolyte, your wise kidneys will direct the excess out of your body. No worries about overdoing it.

Hiking For Her's Trail Food Additional Information

These articles on the HFH website will provide additional information about your day hiking food choices.

Best Trail Snacks

Best Dayhike Foods: Ideas To Make Your Day

Dayhike Food Safety

How To Maintain Hiking Energy

Hiking Nutrition: What You Need To Know

Hiking Calories: Food In, Energy Out

Chapter 4: Hiking Hydration

At home, you drink when you feel thirsty, but is that good enough for the trail?

Find out about hiking water and dehydration in this chapter:

-Water: a nutrient for muscle cells

-Water bottles -vs- hydration systems: pros and cons

-Spot – and fix – dehydration before it robs you of energy

-Sports drinks -vs- plain water

-Electrolyte additions: when to use them

-In praise of perspiration

HIKING WATER AS A NUTRIENT

Drinking water on a hike is common sense, rooted in your everyday awareness of feeling thirsty. But what's the big fuss about *hiking water*?

There are three ways to look at hiking water: through the lens of basic chemistry, in terms of cell biology, or as a hiking impediment on the trail.

If you look at this amazing clear, refreshing fluid as a **chemist,** you see a molecule composed of two hydrogen atoms bonded to an oxygen atom.

This simple arrangement confers **remarkable properties** of heat storage, solubility and dissociation. Planet Earth relies on these properties to maintain its temperature and water balance, which pays off for hikers as we enjoy the seasons.

You can also view water through a **biology lens**: You have to *replace what you lose* via respiration, perspiration, urination, and defecation. Water loss pulls important ions such as sodium and potassium out of your cells, so you need to replenish these **electrolytes** before your body complains (cramps, for instance).

Food intake is one way to replenish; but hikers might need even more help to re-balance (more on that in a moment).

And finally, on a hike, you might regard water as **an obstacle**: streams to wade through, big juicy mud puddles to avoid, knee deep rivers to ford, and my personal favorite: solid and/or liquid precipitation pelting you in the face.

So there's no getting away from water.

For now, let's follow the cell biology route. Specifically, let's look at how to maintain and monitor your water balance during a hike.

Water amounts on a hike

Staying well hydrated on a hike should be a simple matter of drinking when you feel thirsty, right? Sorry, no.

Often, by the time you "feel" thirsty, you've already lost a lot of water via perspiration and respiration. Perfect example: open mouth breathing as you navigate an up-slope on a warm, sunny day.

Short term, not having enough water in your body makes your heart work harder.

Allowing yourself to become dehydrated also sets you up for dehydration headaches and next day hiking inflammation.

To stay well hydrated, you should stop regularly (say, every 45 - 60 minutes) for a water break during a hike. Carrying a water bottle on an exterior pocket of your pack (See Chapter 1) makes it easy to access your water supply.

Regular water breaks also allow you to check the map and stretch a bit.

This "water break habit" leads to deeper mindfulness of the relationship between your body and the trail. And it's the perfect excuse for a carbohydrate-rich (see Chapter 3) snack!

Tip: Too much water hitting an empty stomach quickly makes you feel nauseated, and can lead to "stomach" cramping. Slow and steady sips work best, especially if the water is icy cold and you haven't eaten recently.

Plastic water bottles are lightweight and easy to monitor for fullness. BPA-free plastic is the industry standard, so toss your old plastic bottles and get some new ones.

Tip: Buy one that has the lid attached to the bottle. These are a bit tricky to drink out of, but you'll never have to watch the lid roll downhill.

Tip: Skip the lids with a built in pop up straw because they are hard to clean and will harbor microbes and food debris after a few hikes.

Not a fan of plastic? Metal water bottles are inert, meaning they can't react to anything you put inside of them to create weird tastes. But they are a bit heavier, and will dent if dropped on a rock.

And for cold weather hikes, you might find it unpleasant to put your lips on the metal rim.

See Chapter 4 Resources for some water bottle brands to rely on.

If the idea of stopping for water breaks hurts your soul, you can carry a hydration system (water bladders or reservoirs).

A hiking hydration backpack provides ample room for a full water bladder. Thin plastic tubing brings water from the plastic bladder to your mouth, with a "bite valve" controlling the flow of water.

These hydration systems carry additional responsibilities regarding cleanliness and maintenance, and seem pricey when compared to the price of a water bottle because you need to replace the components when they wear out or crack.

And here's why you might want to think long and hard about using one: It's impossible to gauge how much water you're ingesting, so you might under-hydrate and set yourself up for a headache later.

There's the flip side, too: you consume all of your water half way through the hike, not realizing that you needed to pace yourself.

Regardless of the delivery system, you **need lots of clean water** while you hike, and before and after you hike, too.

With every breath and drop of sweat, water molecules are leaving your body. And don't forget to factor in water lost to urine and feces.

For a day hike, one liter of water is the minimum amount you should carry. In warm weather, two liters provides a nice safety margin in case you're delayed on the trail.

Be sure your pack has outside pockets for two one-liter bottles, or that your hydration bladder is big enough to transport lots of water.

Undeniable hiking fact: Water is heavy. Dehydrated water would be really cool, right?

But having extra water along for a hike gives you that extra margin of safety Chapter 2 was all about. Don't short yourself on water just because it makes your pack heavier.

One more consideration for your water balance: If you consumed dehydrating beverages recently, you are **starting off your hike with a *water deficit*.** Need some examples?

-Morning coffee or tea on the drive to the trail head.

-Last night's beer or carbonated drinks.

-And did you consume salty foods with those beverages?

Heads up: You will need to carry extra water on your hike to avoid a headache and satisfy your thirst sensations if you're starting off a little under-hydrated.

Here's another issue many hikers face: **not feeling thirsty**. Could it be that you've learned to ignore your thirst sensations?

To test this hypothesis, gather together 6 pennies (or quarters, if you're a high roller). Tomorrow morning, put them on your kitchen windowsill or on the edge of your work desk.

-Every time you drink a glass of water, take one of the coins away (add them to your hiking gear fund). Coffee, soda drinks, smoothies – those don't count, and in fact, you should add a coin!

-If you still have coins left at the end of your day, you probably do ignore the subtle signals your brain is sending to your conscious mind.

Monitoring your hydration levels

Here's an easy way to monitor your water level on the trail, other than your thirst: Keep an eye on how much, and what color, you are urinating.

Scant amounts of darkly colored urine are an indication that your kidneys are reclaiming most available water molecules and putting them back into your bloodstream, rather than your urine. Long term, that's not a good plan.

Trail tip: If your trip to the bushes resulted in a little bit of dark urine, drink more water immediately. Monitor the amount and color of your urine at the next pit stop, and drink more water until your urine becomes abundant and pale yellow.

This is especially important if you feel light headed or woozy.

Don't like squatting to pee in the bushes or behind a rock? Try a female urination device! See Chapter 4 Resources for an explanation.

It's never a good idea to avoid urinating. If you've ever had a urinary bladder or kidney infection, you will be nodding your head in agreement. So do what it takes to get comfortable with the idea of taking regular pee breaks.

Another clue to dehydration: a pounding headache that throbs around the temples and pulls at your eyes. You might need to drink a quart or two of water before it goes away, so get started on that right away before the headache escalates.

Popping some pain relief won't undo the fact that you're dehydrated, so begin to drink water before you reach for the ibuprofen.

Best hydration practice after a strenuous hike: Make time to sit quietly and drink at least a quart of pure water, headache or no headache.

If you don't need the water, no harm done - your kidneys will produce abundant clear urine and cells will be properly hydrated. (Kidneys are very wise organs!)

Safe drinking water

How do you know your hiking water is safe to drink?

If it's coming from your water supply at home (most likely scenario for dayhikers), no worries.

But what if you have to resupply during your hike?

There is no way to look at water and know if it's fit to drink. Some of the most pristine, clear water could be carrying microscopic trouble makers.

And just for the record, waterborne hiking illness is no joke.

Refilling your clean hiking water bottles with contaminated water could leave you with very unpleasant, debilitating giardia symptoms.

So play it safe by using the water purification tips on the HFH website. Start with the reviews of two types of Lifestraw products.

Types of hiking water

What should you swallow to keep your body hydrated throughout a hike? Your choices include plain water (either tap or filtered), sports drinks, or enhanced "turbo" water .

For a short day hike in moderate temperatures, **unadulterated tap water** should suffice. You'll get sodium and other electrolytes via your food, and you probably aren't sweating enough to deplete them to a significant (as in muscle cramps or spasms) level.

Filtered water removes some of the minerals, which could affect the taste: "flat" water.

So if your taste buds crave "a little something", you could pack a bottle of **unsweetened flavored, non-carbonated water**.

Why no carbonation? Because it's harder for your body to handle fizzy CO_2 while you're working hard. You are already breathing hard and off-gassing the carbon dioxide waste products of respiration.

Who needs to burp her way down the trail? (Let's leave that one alone, shall we?)

Some of these "**enhanced** waters" boast vitamins to keep you fueled. But do you need those?

B vitamins do help the nervous system do its important work of communicating with your muscles, and are water soluble along with vitamin C. That means with every sip, you're getting the vitamins delivered to your bloodstream.

If you feel better drinking this vitamin enhanced water, carry on!

What about those brightly colored, well marketed **sports drinks** for athletes? Endurance in a bottle!

While it's true that you're an endurance athlete, you probably aren't going to be doing an extreme mileage/elevation hike in just one day.

If you are, then consider Gatorade or some other sports drink.

Drinking water containing electrolytes can keep your muscles going strong, due to the ready supply of ions flowing to your cells. Muscle contractions rely on these ions to generate power strokes; the "electro" in the name indicates that they carry an electrical charge which cell membranes use to do work.

Tip: These convenient bottles of sports drinks contain chemicals to achieve the shocking bright color, and preservatives to extend shelf life, along with a healthy dose of salt and sugar. Do you want to pay for those additions?

Why not add your own electrolytes to your water bottle? That way you can control the amount, quality, and price of these additives.

If that approach sounds good to you, here are a few tips on how to **make your own "turbo" water**:

*Packets of electrolytes are preferred on the trail, rather than adding them to your water bottle before you start.

Two reasons for that: If you buy a large canister and use it slowly, the electrolyte powder tends to get a bit "grainy" and hard to dissolve. Plus, the packets are super convenient to carry.

Stash a few extra packets in your first aid kit (Chapter 2, Ten Essentials) for dehydrated trail buddies, or to use on the days when you forget to toss them into your lunch sack.

*If cost is your primary concern, buy a large canister and write the date of purchase on it. Make it a priority to use it up as quickly as possible. Give it a good shake before scooping out the amount you need.

*Buying electrolytes in bulk guarantees cost savings. Watch for sales, and stock up then.

*Not sure which flavor you'd enjoy most? Purchase a packet of each flavor. Mix up a bottle and sip it during strenuous yard work or after your daily walk. You'll quickly find out which ones you prefer. Why get stuck drinking something unpalatable on your day hike? Chances are, if it tastes bad to you, your hydration level will drop.

*Putting electrolytes into your water bottle or hydration bladder will lead to unwanted microbial growth if it sits for longer than a day. After your hike, wash and rinse your bottle/bladder very thoroughly. Trust me, you don't want the black gunky stuff that blooms if you forget to do this.

*See Chapter 4 Resources for some electrolyte powder brands to try.

Perspiration: it's a good thing.

No, really!

Does that go against what you've been taught in terms of personal hygiene? Think again, dear hiker!

You perspire to dump excess heat in your core. If you're burning up the trail, you don't want your internal organs to get overheated and cease to function, do you? Of course not!

And if you're hiking with a doggie friend, be aware that the only way she can dump excess heat is to pant - which makes her thirsty, which means you've got to carry enough water (or have her carry enough water) to replace what's lost in the drool.

Luckily, you don't need to drool to cool yourself down (although it's an option if you meet a creepy stranger on the trail – see Chapter 6).

Instead, your skin pores open up and release heat trapped in water: sweat, it's called. Perspiration, if you want to get fancy.

Did you realize that working up a good sweat is an age old cleansing technique? Your skin benefits from opening up those pores and flushing them out, so why get in the way of all that goodness?

Oh, wait. Are you offended by the idea of body odor?

Sweat won't smell bad until your normal skin bacteria have had a chance to start metabolizing it, so on a day hike, what you're probably smelling is a person's characteristic "signature" odor.

For example: A garlic eater will have different odor than a curry eater. A meat eater will smell differently than a vegan.

So here's the point: As long as you shower or bathe within hours after a hike, extreme body odor won't be much of a problem.

Maybe you've never really smelled your own signature smell. Here's your chance! Defy the cosmetic and perfume industries, and take a whiff of your own sweaty skin.

How much sweat is "too much"?

Don't ask me. I always have a soaked shirt (see Soaked Shirt Rule, Chapter 10) by the time I reach my destination. Because of this, it's wise to carry a clean, dry shirt to change into at turn-around time (Chapter 5).

If the weather is cool, this simple shirt habit prevents odor buildup as well as hypothermia.

And on a sunny warm day, what fun it is to dry off in the sun - a perfect excuse for an after-lunch siesta.

Can you tell that I'm a big fan of perspiration? It's Mother Nature's way of keeping you cool and clean, inside and out.

Full disclosure: I don't wear antiperspirant or deodorant when I hike, because I want to capitalize on the ability of my sweat to carry away impurities and toxins and to clean out my pores. Try it!

Tip: An additional benefit of muscular contractions during a hike: they get the lymphatic system moving, another way to purify the blood and allow toxins to flow out of the skin pores where they can be flushed away when you shower or swim.

And there's another little known use for perspiration: If you are hiking with someone you are romantically involved with, or *want* to be involved with, the pheromones in your sweat can be a huge turn-on.

Or not.

A lot of human reproduction/romance is tied up in smell. *Really!!* If you don't believe me, ask the perfume manufacturers. They make a fortune on your sense of smell, what you've been taught to accept as a "normal" body odor, and the fact that you perspire.

Ditch the fancy perfumes, and sweat in the general direction of your crush. Good things could happen.

Tip: Use the CONTACT link on the HFH website to invite me to the wedding.

Chapter Four Summed Up.

After reading Chapter 3, you might have thought that food is more important than water on a hike.

Allow me to correct any misconceptions generated by Chapter 3 with this sentence:

Hiking water is vital to efficient cell function, a process that occurs without any conscious thought on your part.

Until your cells start speaking up, that is. Messages from your cells that tell you that you don't have enough water in your bloodstream include muscle spasms, headache, fuzzy thinking, nausea and dark scant urine.

Ignore those little love postcards at your own risk.

A liter of water isn't too much to pack for a dayhike. If it's hot, make that two liters. Think of how strong your legs will be from the additional weight!

Carry water purification tablets or a water filter on long dayhikes, to guarantee that you have a backup plan for abundant quantities of clean water. If this seems like too much work, at least carry an additional quart (a liter would be better) of water in your pack.

The type of water you ingest is a personal decision. The harder you sweat, the more likely you will need to replace electrolytes. Use convenient sports drinks, or add your own to your water bottle.

Sweat early and often! It's good for you. Just be sure to replace all of the water lost to your normal body functions by carrying plenty of the wet stuff.

And stash some water back at the trailhead. Toast to a great dayhike with the wet stuff, and your cells will cheer (listen closely, they really will).

Chapter Four Take-Aways

Water is considered a cellular nutrient, just like carbohydrates, protein and fat covered in Chapter 3.

Carrying a water bottle in the outside pocket of your pack is an inexpensive and reliable way to **monitor your water intake as you hike.**

Hydration systems allow you to sip water throughout your hike. They are expensive, require a firm commitment to good hygiene, and need a backpack that can accommodate the reservoir and tubing.

Sports drinks contain sugar, salt, artificial colors and flavorings along with water, making them expensive and harder to process in your body. They are convenient, though.

Electrolytes can be added to your water if you're really serious about preventing muscle cramps and post-hike aches and pains.

Water in, water out. Monitor the color and amount of urine you produce on a hike. Lots of pale yellow = good. Dark and scarce = bad, so drink up!

Dehydration can show up as a pounding headache at your temples and behind your eyes. Masking the pain with medicine does nothing to restore your water balance. Give your body water to eliminate the underlying problem: lack of water in your bloodstream.

Perspiration means your body is working hard to regulate your internal temperature and clean out your pores. That's a good thing!

Chapter Four Resources

Hiking For Her Hydration Recommendations

ELECTROLYTES

Hiking hydration means keeping the water you put into your body where it belongs: in your body, available to your cells.

In other words, electrolytes help maintain the physiologic balance of your bloodstream so your cells always have the ions (charged particles) they need to do their jobs.

Consider adding powdered electrolytes to your hiking hydration routine in hot or strenuous conditions.

Also, carry a few packets of electrolytes in your first aid kit in case you are losing precious body water via diarrhea or vomiting. It will buy you some time so you can hike out and get help.

I carry Ultima Replenisher packets (love the lemon flavor), which are easy to transport and essentially weightless in your pack.

I have to admit that I look forward to rest stops so I can enjoy the lemony flavor on a hot day. And in the winter, I warm up the water and add the electrolytes before leaving the house. It makes lunch all the more enjoyable: a hot cup of lemony goodness!

The other brand of electrolytes I rely upon is Natural Hydration (Nuun) tablets.

Tablets are lightweight, easy to transport, and super easy to pop into your water bottle.

Just be sure to give them enough time to dissolve, and give your bottle a vigorous shake before you drink.

WATER BOTTLES

I have 2 favorites for water bottles: plastic and metal.

Nalgene is a brand of plastic that has been used in science laboratories for decades. I've been carrying Nalgene for decades, and have no hesitation recommending that you carry a wide mouth, loop topped (BPA free) Nalgene bottle.

Clear plastic bottles are great when you want to see how much water you're drinking at each rest break. And they're not going to dent if you drop them on a rock.

They come in a wide array of colors, too. Colorless is also an option in the Nalgene world.

Metal water bottles are perfect for extra durability and non-reactivity with your electrolytes (no "off" flavors).

I'm a big fan of Klean Kanteen. In fact, I've been carrying Klean Kanteen bottles in 3 sizes for about a decade, and notice they keep water colder for longer than a plastic water bottle in the heat of summer.

Hydroflask is the new kid on the block. Double walled stainless steel insulated water bottle = thermal control over your beverages, year round.

Of course, in the winter, drinking from a cold metal rim is not much fun. That's why I switch back to my Nalgenes for cold weather hiking.

Additional Information on Hydration

Visit the American College of Sports Medicine's website for a free copy of their *Position Stand: Exercise and Fluid Replacement.*

The Natural Hydration Council has Hydration Fact Sheets available, free of charge.

Chapter 5: Destination and Itinerary

Don't rely on luck or hearsay to pick the perfect destination.

In this chapter, you'll learn how to:

-Choose a great destination for your hike

-Find the best maps and other hiking resources

-Leave an itinerary with a trusted person

-Stick to a turn around time

HIKING DESTINATION AND ITINERARY

Your hike actually begins *before* **you leave for the trail head.** No kidding!

The first four chapters of this book have given you ideas for choosing the right gear, food, water and essential trail items for a dayhike.

Now let's turn to selecting a great hiking destination.

To plan a safe and enjoyable hike, you will need to pour over maps of the area you're planning to hike through.

Maps provide data, and data provides a margin of safety:

-how far you'll hike:

-where you can find surface water should you need it,

-what the terrain will be like, and

-possibilities for Plan B in case you get diverted from your original destination.

In the U.S. there are well maintained routes into the wild places near you. How did this wealth of access points accumulate?

Government money was used in the past to build and maintain trails in some locations. In other places, community volunteers and private organizations keep existing trails open while creating new ones. Sometimes, it's a combination of both!

Many foot-only trails exist in an historical context:

-routes to fire towers,

-border patrolling in times of political unrest,

-abandoned mining operations,

-overgrown logging roads,

-mountain climbing access points, and

-fisherman's paths.

If you're a history buff, hunt down the books and documents that tell the tale of the trail! It's a great way to connect personally with the trails you use.

Or perhaps we should take a longer view of historical context. Humans used trails to move seasonally, generation after generation, until the paths became beaten into the earth. Imagine the stories of personal suffering and triumph associated with the hiking trails you use today!

BEST TRAILS FOR DAYHIKING

For beginning day hikers, it's best to pick a trail that is:

-easy to access (paved or well graded roads to established trail heads),

-well marked with no ambiguity at junctions,

-maintained after seasonal storms so blow downs and hazards are removed early in the hiking season,

-of moderate length (less than 10 miles round trip) with modest elevation gain.

As your skill level increases, increase the daily mileage to double digits and tackle more elevation gain per mile.

If you can find a loop hike, so much the better! New scenery for the entire length of the hike is a gift.

So where are you going to find the ideal hike?

Maps, of course.

And where are you going to find the ideal map? Read on!

FINDING THE BEST HIKING TRAIL MAPS

The best hiking maps are easy to use, portable, weather resistant, and in your pack. In other words, they're so great that you should never leave home without one.

You'll be amazed at how quickly your map collection grows as your appetite for outdoor time increases. You know you're addicted when you make a bee line for the map section of your favorite outdoor gear store!

Electronic access to maps has literally opened up a whole universe of hiking options. Let's look at some of your options for acquiring the best hiking trail maps without resorting to a trip to a physical map store.

Free Topographical Hiking Trail Maps

There are plenty of free United States topographical hiking maps, available for instant download thanks to the taxpayers. These maps provide detailed information on contours and land features.

Those details translate into duration and intensity of a hike, which dictate how much time it will take you to reach your turn around point (see below).

Don't leap blindly into a hike without having some idea of how challenging (or snooze worthy) it will be.

Chapter 5 Resources will give you information on how to read a topographical map.

Green Trail Maps

Green Trail maps provide flat maps, folded maps, downloadable maps... but only for a selected few states in the U.S.

However, there's some seriously sweet terrain on these maps, so these little topographical gems deserve a spot in your backpack if you're in an area served by them.

They are indispensable in so many ways:

-finding a surface water source for a quick swim or a water bottle refill,

-converting mileage into estimated arrival time at a turn around spot,

-and my favorite, sitting at a viewpoint and learning the names of the surrounding peaks and drainages.

Always verify recent trail impacts from flash floods or other natural disasters before heading out with one of these maps. They're not updated frequently.

U.S. Forest Service Maps

Inexpensive U.S. Forest Service maps show numbered roads, trails, trail heads, and campgrounds. Use these when you're scoping out an area for the first time, or concentrating your hiking efforts in one locale.

Also use the websites associated with each area to get updated information:

-road closures (fire, flood, downed trees),

-seasonal trail closures (elk mating season), or

-animal activity that might force a trail closure (unruly mountain goats or bears, for example).

You can also cross reference the numbered trails with trail reports posted by bloggers or outdoor organizations that cover your area.

Be sure to check the related website for updated information on the morning of your hike. Things can change fast out there.

Bureau of Land Management (BLM) Maps

The U.S. Department of the Interior (Love that name!! But who's in charge of the exterior??) oversees (and I quote):

-energy

-fire

-grazing

-planning

-recreation

-national conservation lands

-wild horses and burros

-sage grouse conservation

-and a lot of other stuff including noxious weeds.

Whew! That's a lot of overseeing.

BLM also has free maps that you can use to plan some great backcountry dayhikes.

You'll have to poke around a bit to get to the state, and the area within that state, that you're interested in. But again, prepare to get lost in a wealth of free and low cost information.

State Forest Maps

These are super easy to navigate in three easy steps:

Pick a state.

Put that state's name in front of the words "Department of Natural Resources", using your favorite search engine.

Locate some great info, including maps, about hiking opportunities. You just might learn a few new things about an area you thought you knew well.

National Park Hiking Trail Maps

How many national parks are there in the United States?

Ha! Trick question! (Sorry)

If you count everything with a "national" in front of it, there are around 390. But not all of these are good for hiking.

National monuments and national historic sites, for example, aren't going to give you much mileage for a dayhike.

To narrow your options, focus on National Parks (capital P) and the number drops to "only" 60.

So much information! So many trails! And so little time... sigh.

Satellite Image Maps

Why not use the highest level of technology available to plan your next hiking adventure? As in satellite imagery!

These maps are so fascinating! You can pick your location, zoom in and out, build a pretty decent three dimensional representation of an area, and scope out some great destinations.

This is also a great tool if you're not the best at visualizing where you are on a trail. By looking at the route ahead of time, you can begin to build a mental map of the area.

Chapter 7 will explain why that's an important skill for a hiker.

Ready for even more fun? Explore Flash Earth!

National Map Viewer and Download Platform

Since you're geeking around with maps, you might as well try out this site: https://viewer.nationalmap.gov/launch/

It provides the ability to customize a map, adding or subtracting important hiking features such as:

-elevation

-water features

-land cover

-place names

-boundaries

-structures, and

-lots of other things a hiker might like to see (or avoid).

Map reading does take a certain skill set, there's no doubt about it.

If you're going to stray at all from the trail, you need to know how to navigate using a map and compass. Chapter 7 explains why relying on electronic devices isn't such a great idea when you go off-trail.

When you "read" a map, it's not like reading a book. Numbers and little drawings mean a whole lot more than words.

For instance: What scale of map are you talking about?

And what do the hiking trail map symbols mean? More importantly, why would a hiker care?

Luckily, there are free resources waiting for you. Try my links on the HFH website to trustworthy guides to locate, ponder, and utilize maps of the best hiking trails.

But wait! You're sitting there thinking "I'm not a map person. Maps are boring."

Two ways you can go with this (a small map joke, please forgive):

-Always and forever hike with a map lover.

-Grit your teeth and use a map.

Investing a bit of time BEFORE you hit the trail will yield amazing dividends ON the trail - and just might lead to a map addiction! Don't say I didn't warn you.

If you keep at this hiking thing, you're gonna need to build a **map annex** on your abode!

A few map tips before we move on to the importance of a hiking itinerary:

*Always confirm your location at trail junctions by pulling out your map. Don't rely on signage because it might not be there when you need it, or it might not reflect re-routed or newly named trails.

*Carry your maps in a ziplocked waterproof map case, or at least a plastic bag. This protects the paper from not only water but trail dirt, hungry rodents and careless trail buddies.

*Want to get really serious? Laminate your maps at an office supply store.

*As you hike more and more often through your favorite areas, try to build a mental map of the locale. Confirm your mental map by putting your small maps together to build an overview of what your hiking area looks like from a bird's eye view. Then check your understanding using the satellite imagery mentioned above.

*When resting at a lofty viewpoint, practice your mental map skills. For example, how would you represent the distance to nearest ridge line, compared with a distant lake?

These mental skills might also come in handy in your non-trail life.

At the very least, you will be aware of where you are in your surroundings, and that's no small thing for a hiker.

LEAVE AN ITINERARY

Let's borrow this concept from the travel industry to keep you safe on the trail.

And let's keep it short and sweet: Someone you trust needs to know where you went, what time you will return, and what to do if you don't show up on time.

Why not have a standing arrangement with a neighbor, friend or family member? Text or email them the info below.

-The car's make, model, color and license plate number that brought you to the trail head (don't assume they already know this if it's your car)

-Your destination, including where the trail head is, name and number of the trail, direction of travel, expected mileage, and any other details such as name of National Forest or Forest Service road number

-Your estimated start and end times

-Your cell phone number

-Who you will be hiking with and their phone numbers.

All of this information will be required to get a search and rescue effort started, in case things don't go as planned.

Having this itinerary in hand will take some of the stress out of this process for those back home who are wondering where the heck you are.

Tip: In my experience, a quick phone call or verbal exchange isn't reliable. Details can be forgotten, names of destinations can be mis-remembered – all of which will create confusion for searchers.

Include plenty of details in your written message to your trusted itinerary holder.

Tip: Have a Plan B sketched out, just in case trail conditions or road closures make you bail on your original plan. Note this Plan B in your itinerary. If possible, text your trusted person back home when you switch into Plan B mode.

And to close the loop, be sure to contact him/her when you're safely back home again. Failing to do this might result in a severe tongue lashing, and you'll probably have to find a new itinerary holder.

TURN AROUND TIME: NON-NEGOTIABLE

Please don't be the hiker who asks everyone (s)he meets on the trail "How much farther?" and "What time is it?"

These unprepared day hikers are accidents waiting to happen, because they have no clue where they are or how many hours of daylight they have left to get back to the trail head in one piece.

You, however, are smarter than that. You know that to establish a firm turn around time gives you a wide margin of safety on your day hike, just in case something goes wrong and you need extra time.

Use this six step action plan to create that margin of safety for yourself. This is especially critical if you are hiking solo.

Step One: Figure out **how many miles or kilometers** lie between the trail head and your objective (waterfall, viewpoint, or lunch spot). This is a cinch, given your insatiable appetite for maps (see above).

Step Two: Get a rough idea of the **topography** of your hike, using topo maps, Google Earth, on line hiking trip reports, or any other resource you can find. You got this information earlier in this chapter, and you will use this information in Step 5.

Step Three: Decide on an **arrival time** at the trail head. Factor in local traffic patterns, day of the week (crowded weekend trail heads versus the solitude of Monday morning), whether you will travel on fast highways or two lane roads, etc.

Step Four: Factor in **seasonal and weather conditions**. You'll want to take things easy in the long daylight hours of extreme heat, but will be more inclined to zoom along on a cool, crisp spring day when the sun sets early.

Step Five: Assume you can hike at least **two miles per hour for a flat trail**. Notch this number downward if you're doing a lot of elevation gain/loss. You can always pleasantly surprise yourself with an early arrival at your destination, thus granting yourself extra lounging, photography, journaling or exploring time.

Step Six: **Do the math!** But *do it twice*.

Run the numbers the first time **at home**, the day you finalize which trail you'll be using.

Write down your expected arrival time at the trailhead, round trip mileage*, hiking pace based on expected trail conditions, and approximate time of twilight.

Weather related note: Darkness falls early on cloudy stormy days, so check weather forecasts before you actually leave for the trailhead. You might have to adjust your numbers a bit.

Hiking in dense forests? Early twilight needs to be factored in. (You are carrying your headlamp, as Chapter 2 suggested, right?)

Also factor in how much time you want for breaks, seeing the sights, and a lunch stop. This data allows you to figure out when you need to start turning around in order to get back to the trailhead without using a faster pace than necessary (see Chapter 8).

*A round trip mileage number might be inaccurate for calculating your pace for a couple of reasons. The way out always seems shorter because you're already aware of navigational challenges like tree blow downs or trail detours; you won't have to stop and figure things out. On the flip side, your legs are more tired on the way out so your pace might slow down.

The second time? Do the math **on the trail.** Keep track of exact times with your cell phone's timing feature: turn it on as you step onto the trail, and turn it off when you're taking off your boots back at the trailhead.

Then compare your estimate with your actual time. How far off were you? Use this data to learn how to become a better estimator of turn around time.

Tip: If you need to be the turn around time "enforcer" in your hiking group, stand firm. There is no Hiking Hall of Shame for hikers who turn around without achieving an objective.

But there should be one for hikers who push beyond the bounds of sanity and end up needing the services of the local Search & Rescue team.

Also note that some day hikers love to push the envelope, thinking nothing of hiking back to the trail head via head lamp or flash light.

If that idea gives you the heebie jeebies, make it abundantly clear that the turn around time in non-negotiable.

This prevents the dilemma of "should I turn around by myself?" from rearing its ugly head. A group of hikers need to stay together, or find new hiking partners (see Chapter 10).

Chapter Five Summed Up

Pretty basic stuff in this chapter, but that doesn't mean it isn't critical for keeping yourself safe on the trail.

Plus, hiking maps bring new meaning to the phrase *"happy trails"*.

Find a map and use it to plan your hike. This chapter gave you abundant free and low cost map resources.

Carry a map with you during your hike.

Practice using a map until it becomes second nature to pull it out and confirm your position at trail junctions or areas where the trail gets a little sketchy.

Don't leave for the trailhead without leaving your hiking plans with at least one other person back home. This is absolutely critical, each and every time, if you're a solo hiker.

And always have a Plan B in your back pocket. If nothing else, Plan B can become the next hike you do!

A turn around time is notoriously important for mountain climbers. Use that same discipline as a dayhiker, and never have to say you're sorry to the Search And Rescue team.

Chapter Five Take-Aways

Always have a **set destination** in mind for your dayhike.

Follow **established trails** which are **clearly marked** on your map.

Carry the appropriate **topographical maps**, and consult them frequently to identify landmarks and trail junctions.

Don't hike without at least one other non-hiking person having your **written itinerary**.

Establish your **turn around time** ahead of time, and stick to it.

Chapter Five Resources

Hiking For Her's Additional Information

MAPS:

National Geographic provides a 32 page pdf instant download booklet, entitled Basic Map and GPS Skills

Visit Map My Hike.

http://www.topozone.com gives away topographical maps of the United States

https://dzjow.com/2012/04/12/free-online-topographic-maps-for-hiking/ offers topo maps for the world!

TRAILS:

Visit the HFH website for these articles:

Best Hiking Trails

Hiking Trail Maps

Topographical Maps For Hikers

Hiking Map Scales And How To Use Them

Hiking Map Symbols: A Fun Language

More online resources:

Check americantrails.org/resources/statetrails for trails in the United States.

For Canadian trails, go here: canadatrails.ca/hiking

During Your Hike

If you don't feel safe, turn around.

If it's not fun, stop hiking and figure out why!

This section is all about how to make your hikes memorable for the right reasons.

Chapter 6: Safety and Comfort

Chapter 7: Navigation

Chapter 8: Pacing

Chapter 6: Safety and Comfort

Chapter 6 shows you how to handle mental and physical trail issues with ease and confidence, including:

-Trailhead awareness

-Strangers on the trail

-Animal encounters

-Creepy crawlies

-Basic weather smarts

-Emergencies and injury

-Blisters

-Female trail hygiene

Good hikers also care about the safety and comfort of other trail users. Etiquette and ethics are subjects that aren't discussed much, but should be.

Chapter 6 will conclude by giving you the goods on how to be a good citizen on the trail:

-Trail etiquette

-Leave No Trace (LNT) principles

TRAIL SAFETY

Trail safety for women hikers involves using your head once you begin your hike.

It's all about *knowing*, as in knowing some of the things already covered:

-what you can use in your pack when trouble pops up (Ten Essentials, Chapter 2)

-where you are throughout the hike (Maps, Chapter 5)

-which terrain, distance and elevation gain suits you best, (Planning, Chapter 5)

-and when to turn around (Chapter 5).

But now it's time to hit the trail.

Chapter 6 gives you what you need to stay not only safe, but comfortable and confident during your day hike.

Safety + comfort = an enjoyable hike!

Let's start at the beginning of your dayhike: your arrival at the trailhead.

TRAILHEAD BEST PRACTICES

You know exactly where the trailhead is, because you read Chapter 5 and have chosen a great dayhike destination.

But maybe you've never actually seen the trailhead, or driven on the roads leading to it.

Given this unfamiliarity, budget in some extra time to get there. This is especially true for travel on unpaved or minimally maintained roads such as Forest Service or county roads.

If at all possible, check on line for **road closures** and **seasonal problems** such as washouts or forest fires. If the area has experienced severe weather recently, odds are good that the types of roads hiker rely upon will be affected.

If your vehicle has low clearance, you will find yourself slowing to a crawl to navigate pot holes, washboard surfaces, fallen tree limbs, deep mud puddles, rock fall and more.

You might also need **parking permits**. These permits usually aren't available at the trailhead, and you risk tickets and fines if you ignore them. No parking permit means you will have to abort your hiking plans, or backtrack to the latest permit dispensing building.

Once you reach the trailhead, verify that it's the right one by double checking your map or looking for signage. If things don't line up with your expectations, pull out your map(s) and figure it out.

Scope out the **best parking place** for your vehicle: near the outhouse, or furthest away? Then decide whether to back in, parallel park, or other types of parking that make the most sense for the configurations of the area.

If given the choice, always turn your car to face toward the way out. This eliminates getting boxed into tight spaces by cars arriving later in the day.

Be a good citizen by not boxing in others!

If you're dayhiking alone, be aware of who else is at the trailhead when you arrive. Do a gut check or use your spidey senses (Chapter 2: additions to Ten Essentials) to size up anyone who appears to be lingering, loitering or lurking.

A real dayhiker is businesslike, putting on boots and pack, checking a map, eating a snack. A lurker stands out because… well, you know why.

What to do if you feel uncomfortable about walking away from your vehicle? Don't! Get back inside, and make it look like you're searching for an item in your pack, checking your phone, or reading trail directions.

If after 5 minutes the lurker is still not acting like a hiker, you might want to try a different trail head. Which is not a problem, since you worked Plan B into your itinerary, right? (Chapter 5)

Assuming you feel comfortable about getting out of your vehicle, there are a few things you can do to get your dayhike started on the right note.

-Take a few sips of water from the extra water container you stowed in your vehicle. You didn't think the "extra water"(Chapter 2) rule applied only to the trail, did you?

-Do a few stretches (Chapter 9) to warm up your muscles.

-Double check where you stowed your car keys. If your daypack has a clip inside one of the pockets, use it to securely clip the keys into the pack. Otherwise, stow keys in a zipped pocket in your pants or jacket. Make sure everyone hiking together knows where the keys are, just in case.

-Lace up your boots, but not too tightly. Your feet are going to swell, and you definitely want some wiggle room for your toes as you get into your hiking stride.

-Start off with as few layers of clothing as possible. It's disheartening to have to stop to peel off a jacket or vest after only 5 minutes on the trail. And it completely wrecks your hiking pace (Chapter 8).

-On sunny days, apply sunscreen and UV blocking lip balm at the trailhead. It takes more time than you might think for these to begin working, and they go on better if you're not already a hot, sweaty mess like you will be soon. (Note to self: Hot, sweaty mess is a good thing, in hiker terms!)

-If breakfast is a distant memory, eat a banana or some other fast high carbohydrate snack before setting off.

-Take advantage of any bathroom facilities but always bring your own toilet paper and hand sanitizer because you can't rely on a fully stocked restroom. Lid down when finished, please.

STRANGERS ON THE TRAIL

If you're hiking with someone else, meeting strangers on the trail is no big deal, right? It's an application of the "safety in numbers" rule that every woman intuitively understands (Mother Nature's flocks and herds, too).

A solo dayhiker needs to turn up her gut feelings to full volume, and listen to them. Your gut is giving you free advice.

Popular trails attract social people, so expect to exchange greetings frequently with strangers. The majority of these hikers will not trip your internal stranger danger meter.

If you choose to pass everyone on the trail and remain silent, that's your call. But if you want information about the trail conditions up ahead, a brief chat can supply valuable insight into how your hike is going to unfold.

Advice for any female hiker, solo or not: if something feels or looks wrong about someone you meet on the trail, ask yourself why – and listen to your reasoning. Avoid any self-talk that dismisses this type of information (you know, the "good girl" trap).

Example: If a guy you meet on the trail seems too chatty, stands too close, or is very curious about where you're going, make up a story about your fictitious hiking partners waiting for you. Get away from him without giving away any personal information.

Example: You meet someone who isn't dressed like a hiker, and who acts uncomfortable to see you on the trail. Don't stop to chat, just blast on past him/her. You have my permission to be "rude".

Tips for female hikers:

*If you hike near busy urban areas, consider how to keep yourself safe where non-hikers have easy access to trailheads and campgrounds. Your options include self defense maneuvers, a canine companion large enough to appear intimidating, pepper spray/mace, or a weapon. Take classes and be prepared for the consequences of your decision and actions. Be especially vigilant about how your selected option could be used against you.

*Project an aura of self confidence on the trail: Stand tall, make eye contact, avoid looking uncertain or hesitant.

*Never look like an easy target. Avoid these "victim" actions: head down and absorbed in checking your phone, not knowing where you are or where you're headed, acting overly friendly or helpful when someone requests information or help from you.

*Explore the fine line between caution and fear, and always listen to your vibes. Don't have any vibes? You've been suppressing them. Let them out of their dark, cramped closet and put them to work for you on the trail.

ANIMAL ENCOUNTERS OF THE LARGE KIND

If you are hiking with at least one other person, your chances of spotting anything larger than a rodent are pretty spotty.

Human voices carry over long distances, so trail chit chat and the noise of your feet and poles will announce your presence to the local wildlife.

Tip: If hiking solo, use this fact to your advantage to become aware of noisy approaching hikers. You can decide if you want to step off the trail and let them pass without seeing you, or if you want to exchange greetings.

Realize that the sound of rushing water or gusts of wind will hide your presence from the local inhabitants. If you've done some advance reading about the area, you'll know which large mammals make it their home turf.

Bears are active at any time of the day or night, and tend to roam around looking for food. They use trails as easy access to water, meadows and other places that hikers like to enjoy.

When hiking through known brown bear territory, carry bear spray and know how and when to deploy it.

Make noise to alert any bear that you're passing through his/her living room, especially when hiking around noisy water features.

If you see bear cubs, immediately back track as fast as you can and abandon the trail to mama bear. This situation can quickly escalate into a confrontation that you do not want to have. Chapter 6 Resources give you more information.

Should you be scared of meeting a cougar on the trail? Only solo hikers should be truly concerned about going up against a big cat.

Cougars (mountain lions) tend to be most active when dayhikers aren't on the trail: early morning or dusk. And their secretive nature keeps them hidden and silent, even when you hike past them.

Again, the resources at the end of this chapter give you more details.

A note about snake encounters: Snakes would much prefer to avoid you. In fact, rattlers give you plenty of warning so you can do the right thing: back away slowly and avoiding shrieking in fear until you're well away from the snake.

Don't be careless with your feet and hands at rest stops or pit stops (pee breaks). Use your hiking poles (Chapter 1) to investigate a place that you're going to sit.

Rattlesnakes are masters of camouflage, so scan and/or probe the area a couple of times before you sit down, put down your pack, or scramble off trail.

It's always wise to know ahead of time the types of snakes you are likely to encounter. At the very least, look at photos of the poisonous ones, so you don't go into freak out mode for no reason when a generic snake slithers across the trail.

A few general tips regarding wildlife encounters on a dayhike:

*Watch for signs of large mammal activity along the trail, such as scratches and claw marks on a tree that are off the ground.

The higher up on the tree, the larger the animal. Fresh marks are easy to spot, because the tree sap will "weep" and draw your eye to it.

*Listen for movement in the areas bordering the trail: breaking branches, rocks rolling downhill, or vocalizations by the animals as they communicate with their offspring.

*Bears like to wallow, and to take naps in cool, shaded areas. If you see prints in the mud around surface water, you're in the bear's living room (which can be a huge area).

If you see compressed grasses or a scruffed up patch beneath a tree, you're in its bedroom!

*While you will probably never see a cougar, you might stumble upon a fresh kill that a cat will defend: a carcass with dirt kicked over the top.

Ravens and other scavengers might help you notice it, with their noisy activity. Pay attention when birds and animals take an interest in a pile of dirt!

Your response: walk out of the area quickly, but never run (it triggers the predator-prey response, exactly what you don't want to do). If possible, don't turn your back on the carcass.

If the cat appears, don't make eye contact. Keep backing away while facing the cat, trying to look as fearsome and large as possible.

Use your voice to tell the cat that you're a scrawny human! Or recite poetry. Just make yourself look and sound like a two legged non-deer.

CREEPY CRAWLIES

Sad as it is for this nature lover to admit, insect repellents might be an important part of your hiking repertoire.

And why do we, sturdy and resolute hikers, want to **repel insects**? Seriously, aren't we outdoors to soak up the *full* Nature experience?

The answer depends upon the hiker you're asking. Beauty, and loathing, are in the eye of the beholder.

Some hikers are deathly afraid of bees and other stinging insects. Allergies, pain, or simply not understanding what the insect is doing as it buzzes around can lead to deep seated phobias that get reinforced on the hiking trail.

And don't think this issue won't come up if you're all hunky dory about insects. If you're hiking with a person who has insect phobias, it can lead to an unpleasant trail experience when that person transforms into a wailing, flailing freak out right in front of your eyes.

Tip: It's probably a good idea to ask your hiking partners about insect issues, if you haven't already. That way you won't be caught off guard (or wounded accidentally) by a flying hiking pole.

Another reason for repellents is to minimize exposure to disease. There are certain insects (mosquitoes) and other small biting trouble makers (ticks) which act as vectors, transferring diseases to humans in their saliva.

Examples of these diseases in the United States include Lyme (Borreliosis) disease, West Nile fever, and encephalitis.

The Zika virus also is in the news lately, and working its way northward into the United States. This one deserves attention from women of child bearing age, as it targets fetal development.

One other reason to repel insects: insect bites hurt or itch, taking your focus off the trail. And if you scratch them with your dirty nails (unavoidable on the trail), you can set yourself up for a secondary bacterial skin infection.

Now that we've reviewed the reasons to repel, let's cover how to do the repelling.

Effective insect repellents

So what should you rely on to repel insects?

You have some choices, and you need to be clear about the pros and cons of each choice. All insect repellents are NOT alike.

First choice: widely available, inexpensive chemicals that affect the insects in various ways.

DEET is the classic example of a manufactured insect repellent. It was developed by the U.S. military, and is now widely available in various strengths. It can be applied to skin, to clothing, or both.

Why does it work? Insects can't stand the way it tastes! Which is the first clue that it might be toxic. And in fact, it does inhibit a key enzyme in mammalian central nervous systems.

You're a mammal, so you need to be cautious with your applications of this chemical, and avoid using it on very young kids whose nervous systems are still developing.

A little of this stuff goes a long way. Be mindful of how much you are applying to your skin, and be sure you can't avoid insects in some other way before you use DEET.

Another chemical name you may have seen: permethrin. It's used to kill ticks and repel insects.

This is another heavy duty chemical, toxic to cats and fish, but not dogs (good to know if your canine companion licks your hand).

Use it carefully on your clothing, and be aware that it is considered a carcinogen.

I've used both of these chemicals in Alaska, Greenland and the Canadian Rockies: hot spots for insects. But sparingly, ever so sparingly ... which is a good rule to follow.

Only use them when you must, and only use the minimal amount to do the job.

Natural insect repellents

To avoid chemical toxicities, you might be interested in natural insect repellents.

I always carry a small bottle of Neem oil with me, to use not only to avoid bites but to take away the swelling and itchiness afterwards (if I forget to apply it before setting off on a hike).

So what is Neem? It's a vegetable oil made from an evergreen tree which grows in India. It's not meant to be ingested, but applied to the skin.

It has a unique odor, which I find hard to describe. Not exactly unpleasant, but definitely noticeable. If you have a super sensitive nose, be forewarned.

It doesn't work 100% of the time, but it's effective enough to avoid chemical exposures in some situations. See if it works for you!

There are other natural repellents on the market that you should consider. Chapter 6 Resources will give you details.

Bug nets

In extremely buggy areas, bug nets that you wear on your face, hands, or body are a life saver. There are advantages and drawbacks to hiking inside of these nets.

Advantages:

1. Cheap! $10 or so for fine mesh netting that you throw on over your hat, and you're good to go. The price goes up for larger nets, but run the cost-benefit analysis and then decide if you need a net.

2. Negligible weight in your pocket, or on your body.

3. Cinches down for a reasonably good custom fit, depending on what else you're wearing.

4. The net comes with a very portable stuff sack for easy storage inside your pack, but could easily be overlooked or thrown out as you empty your pockets (thus becoming a "con").

Disadvantages:

1. Difficult to eat and drink while wearing! You need to quickly lift the net, gulp your beverage or food, and make sure the little bloodsuckers aren't inside the net with you as you enjoy your mouthful.

2. Diminished visibility can make navigating the trail a challenge. Everything looks a bit darker even in bright sunlight! This can create problems if you're hiking on a steep slope and need to keep glancing down to maintain your footing.

And if you're having your picture taken, only the netting will be visible – not your charming smile or wry grin.

3. After awhile, the netting feels a bit scratchy on the face and neck if a breeze is blowing it up against your skin.

4. The interior of the net quickly becomes stuffy and warm when the sun is shining. Luckily, mosquitoes tend to disappear in bright sunlight so this may be a non-issue for you.

BASIC WEATHER SMARTS

Safe hiking weather and perfect hiking weather are very much alike:

-blue skies,

-a few puffy white clouds overhead,

-a gentle warm breeze to cool your face,

-and lots of daylight hours to spend on the trail.

Ah! Perfection!

Gray drizzle or low scudding clouds obscuring the mountains, thunderstorms every afternoon in the summer, or sudden snow squalls in July at high elevations are more realistic if you take a lot of hikes.

Add in the probability of high winds, lightning, sudden temperature swings... and hiking safety can get dicey on the trail.

So it pays to know how to hike through any kind of weather pattern. But better yet? Evasive action!

To avoid nasty surprises and be prepared to handle emerging weather, get familiar with the NOAA.gov website.

Tip: I highly recommend looking at this weather site the day before, and the morning of, your hike to give yourself the best shot at anticipating changeable hiking weather conditions.

The beauty of this site, beyond its reliability and accessibility, is that you can type in the location of your hike and get a **local forecast**. (NOTE: North America only).

In addition, you can check **satellite images** of the area and see **weather alerts for extreme conditions** such as wind, heat, storms or flash floods.

And you can get even *geekier on this site!* Check out the wind speed charts, cloud cover projections, and precipitation forecasts that show you 24 hours of likely hiking weather conditions, and even more weather toys!

Once on the trail, you're on your own. But as we saw at the trail head, awareness will keep you alert to potential trouble.

Tip: Stay alert to changes in wind speed and direction. Note what the clouds are up to. Has the temperature changed suddenly?

Here's a specific example. A sudden burst of wind means a pressure system is passing through, possibly bringing trouble in its wake. When you experience a few minutes of wind gusts, ask yourself:

-Do I have a place to take shelter during a down pour?

-Am I in terrain where sudden run off could sweep me away or cut off access to home?

-Do I have my waterproof gear handy?

-Am I under tree limbs which could harm me if they snap in the wind?

-Is it time to assume the "lightning position"?

You can see what I'm getting at, right? Use your knowledge of safe hiking weather to size up the situation and take immediate action to ensure your safety.

Proactive, rather than reactive, is always the wiser approach as a dayhiker.

Another hiking weather example: If you're at higher elevations, be prepared for sudden precipitation - including snow- year round. Watch the skies and know when to take cover (if there is any).

I've been caught in snow in June, July AND August in the northern hemisphere, and if I hadn't been prepared with my ten essentials (Chapter 2), I'd have been miserable or hypothermic.

If you like to hike in dense forest, the weather may get a little hard to read - that's why knowing the forecast (previously discussed) is so important. My advice? If you feel raindrops on your hat, it must be raining :)

Seriously, you need to watch the sky to whatever extent is possible, read the wind, and learn what cloud types mean.

If nothing else, know that high clouds don't usually bring trouble right away, but watch out for those low scudding clouds on the horizon.

Another important environmental clue that you can use on the trail: Animals and birds will help you out with reading the weather, if you pay attention.

Have you ever noticed that the trail gets very quiet before an impending thunder storm? There's very little cross chatter from the birds, and small mammals make themselves scarce. When it gets quiet, you should think about taking cover, or cover up.

Tip: A sudden silence on a forest trail may also mean that a big predator (bear, cougar or human) is heading your way. To be fair, the reverse also holds true: a scolding squirrel (who is safely in a tall tree) will reveal the presence of a land or air predator.

The best defense against wet or windy weather any hiker has is being prepared. Carry appropriate clothing waterproof jacket & pants, gaiters, and hat, as outlined in Chapters 1 and 2.

Tip: Have these items handy in an outside pocket or top compartment of your backpack so you don't waste precious time digging around when you need them. It's a bummer when your other gear (and lunch) gets wet as you dig around frantically inside your pack.

Wild weather conditions are when you will find out the difference between these terms: water repellent, water resistant, and water proof.

You also want to avoid getting your entire pack wet, so carry a pack cover.

Note that some day packs come equipped with a fitted rain cover. For instance, each of my Deuter packs (see Chapter 1) has a rain fly tucked into a zip pocket on the bottom of the pack. The brightly colored cover, made of water repellent fabric, is tethered to the pack so it can't blow off or get lost when I set the pack down.

Check for this optional feature when you're looking at daypacks.

It's OK to use a large trash bag as a pack cover for your first few hikes, but the day will come when you will want a "real" cover that doesn't get hole-y.

Tips for garbage bag users:

*Be sure you carry more than one garbage bag, because they snag and rip open.

*Pay the extra money for the heavy duty variety.

*Duct tape wrapped around your water bottle will help with field repairs.

OK, class, so what's the take home message on safe hiking weather? All together now:

Don't let less-than-ideal weather keep you inside!

Fair weather day hikers miss out on some great experiences. Some of my most memorable animal encounters have been on rain hikes, probably because the big mammals didn't expect humans to be roaming around in the rain.

Believe me when I tell you that with a weather forecast and the proper gear, and most importantly, the proper attitude, you can hike all 4 seasons through everything Mother Nature throws at you.

With a smile on your face, no less.

So do yourself and your trail buddies a favor: Read up on safe hiking weather. If Mother Nature cannot catch you by surprise, your hiking trips will be safer, warmer and drier and probably more adventurous.

You'll also have the trail all to yourself. Most humans prefer to be on the couch in rainy weather. Defy the masses!

Bonus: Cloud watching is very relaxing (until the hail hits).

RESPONDING TO EMERGENCIES AND INJURY

When the unexpected happens, you have to act fast to decide among several choices:

-Send someone for help (not an option for solo hikers).

-Wait for help to arrive, thanks to your itinerary (Chapter 5).

-Get yourself out of trouble and back to the trailhead (Chapter 2, Ten Essentials).

-Do nothing. Does panicking count as nothing?

Any of these choices can induce *major* trail stress. However, these trail stresses can be handled confidently with some advance planning.

Not interested in investing time and energy into taking heavy duty emergency response courses? Most dayhiker probably don't need to be highly trained beyond basic first aid.

But at the very least, read about other hikers who experienced adversity on the trail and came out on top. Chapter 6 Resources will give you some suggestions.

Training, reading, asking yourself "what if?" questions and then finding the answers, all of these actions will fill up your memory banks with facts.

Cold, hard facts take the edge off the free floating anxiety you feel when thinking about potential trail emergencies. This is important, because decisions made from an emotional stance won't be as solid as those based on fact.

Since you can never predict when you will need to get yourself through unexpected trail stress, let's take a look at three of the four options, one at a time. Note: panic is not a viable option.

Granted, it's not much fun to think about what to do when faced with worst case scenarios. But it's something every hiker should face in theory long before having to face it in reality.

Please resist the urge to skip this part of the chapter, and read these good options for when things go awry on the trail.

Trail stress and safety: Option #1

Can you **send for help**, in the form of your trail partner(s)?

This might not have to happen, if you're carrying an electronic device that can indicate your position and situation (Chapter 7). But if the electronics fail you, your hiking buddies can literally come to your rescue by hiking out for help.

If you're solo, are you carrying a personal locator beacon? Read Chapter 7 for reasons why you might want to.

Signaling, or sending a buddy for help, sets the aid wheels in motion.

Help will be on its way sooner or later, but consider the fact that it might be later. This means you must face the possibility of being alone, perhaps overnight or longer.

That's when your ten essentials (Chapter 2) are going to come out of your pack and save you from stress and worry.

You'll have enough to eat and drink, you can start a fire, you have insect repellent and warm clothes, you'll be able to take shelter from the elements, and you'll have pain relief if needed.

Mentally, you will need to be tough with yourself as you wait for help. Worrying will eat into your energy reserves. That's a bad idea in ways that I'm sure you can visualize.

Trust your hiking buddy or personal locator beacon to get help quickly and efficiently, while you get some sleep/rest.

Trail stress and safety: Option #2

Waiting for help until someone realizes that you're missing is your second option.

This scenario unfolds if you're hiking solo without a communication or panic button device. It can also happen when everyone in your hiking group is affected by a weather event.

No worries! You left your itinerary behind, right? (Chapter 5) Thankfully, a responsible "someone" knows which trail head you parked at, which vehicle you arrived in, where you were headed, and any alternative plans you made (Plan B details).

That trustworthy person also knows that you haven't called, texted or emailed to announce your safe completion of the hike.

Now it's up to you to sit tight and let that trusted someone do the right thing.

-Your 10 essentials will get you through.

-Your itinerary will get the rescuers pointed in the right direction.

While you wait, your task is to make yourself highly visible/audible to the searchers. Help them find you by doing these things:

-Locate an open area that you can access to make it easy for someone to spot you. If the weather is foul, stay under cover until you hear or see activity, then move to this open area.

-Try to sleep when it's dark, so you're alert and able to respond in daylight hours to rescue efforts.

-If you have a colorful tarp or vivid piece of clothing, be sure it's prominently displayed to catch a rescue team's attention from the air.

-If you have a whistle, signal mirror or smoke canister, have it ready to use when you hear a plane/helicopter or people calling your name.

As you do the hard work of waiting patiently, avoid beating yourself up mentally. You got into this situation and you will get out.

Patience and calmness are your mental allies, and will keep your physical energy reserves intact for the actual rescue event.

Trail stress and safety: Option #3

Third option:**Get out by yourself.**

I don't recommend rushing away from the spot you find yourself in, unless there's a compelling reason revolving around your safety. Mistakes get made in haste.

If you feel panicked or anxious at all, **SIT DOWN and WAIT** until that shaky feeling passes. You need to have full control over your thought processes before making your move.

First things first: Use the items in your pack (Chapters 1 and 2) to solve your immediate problems of thirst, hunger, coldness and pain.

Someone knows which trail you used, right? Will the world end if you get home late?

You have *all the time in the world* to make the right choice, and you should use that time to think through why you're in such a hellbent hurry.

If you have this little meeting with yourself and you do decide to get back to the trail head under your own power, be very deliberate and smart about it.

Here's how:

-Bring all of your navigational tools and training to bear on this problem. If you're lost, realize that you started the day knowing where you were. You're not that far from the trailhead.

-Wait until you have good visibility and a clear head to begin moving again.

-Double check your bearings frequently, especially if you're tired.

-Keep track of your new landmarks in case you have to backtrack and start over. Use paper and pen to make notes.

-If you become discouraged or completely disoriented, **STOP**. It might be time to fall back on Option 2 (outlined above).

In the United States, most dayhikes are within walking distance of a road, trail or creek that will lead you back to civilization.

Tip: Can you get to a higher vantage point to spot one?

Following water downhill will lead you to a road eventually, unless you are in the extreme back country (a rare event for a dayhiker). Consult your map, locate a stream or lake, and go from there.

Caveat: But only if you really have to move from the area, the weather is clear, and you have lots of daylight and physical strength to work with. Otherwise, stay put to avoid making it harder for Search and Rescue to find you.

Trail stress: one last thought

Let's finish up with an important biological fact.

Hiking is a stress relieving activity. The levels of the stress hormone called *cortisol* circulating in your bloodstream will decrease as you hike.

That's why you feel a bit depleted physically at the end of a hike, yet at peace.

So don't work against yourself and ADD cortisol to your bloodstream by stressing yourself out with no way to deal with unexpected trail events.

Arm yourself ahead of time with knowledge. That's the only way to avoid the anxiety of not knowing what to do.

Ask any prepared, smart, confident trail woman, and I'm sure they'll agree. Time for you to join the club!

BLISTERS

Let's keep this simple: **Blister prevention is better than blister treatment.**

You, an active hiker, do not want blisters. *Trust me on this.*

To prevent the pain and nasty side effects of blisters, use the Hiking For Her approach outlined below.

1. **Spend time and money on finding boots** that fit properly. Keep trying until you find boots that give you no cause for concern on any type of terrain, or any length of hike.

The quest for the holy grail of hiking (great footwear and hiking socks - see Chapter 1) is worth this investment.

2. **Duct tape spots on your feet** that feel hot or tender after the first hour of hiking. Here's how:

-Before heading to the trail, loop a few feet of duct tape around your water bottle. If you use a hydration system rather than a bottle (Chapter 4), wind it around a part of your hiking pole that won't interfere with its function.

-Tear off chunks of tape as needed at your first rest/water break. Even better, take a break when you first notice a hot spot (area of concern, like heel or toes).

-Be sure you don't tape your socks to your feet or the inside of your boots. You want your feet to move freely with each step, yet not slide around or stick to the sides.

-Duct tape doesn't breathe very well, and is slick enough to make you change your stride. It might not be the fix for every hot spot. See Chapter 6 Resources for other ideas.

3. Carry an extra pair of boots or trail shoes in your pack.

I have been known to do this if I don't trust a new or cranky pair of boots. As far as my feet are concerned, the extra weight is worth it for blister prevention.

But it might seem a bit extreme to you. It is an option worth mentioning, though.

4. Play around with different sock combinations.

Liners and hiking socks abound! But not all of them are designed for the type of hiking you like to do. So be willing to experiment until you find exactly what works best for you.

And don't get discouraged. Luckily, socks are not as pricey as boots, and you'll eventually find the perfect boot and sock combo if you keep at it.

One more idea: swap socks (clean ones, of course) with hiking buddies until you chance upon The Magic Combination.

5. Pay attention to your toenails.

Trim your nails before each hike. Get rid of hang nails.

If you notice that you clench your toes inside your boots due to nail issues, it can lead to blisters or worse - hammer toes, for instance. That's an Ouch that will sideline your hiking career for a long time.

6. Know what normal wear & tear looks like on your feet.

Here's a personal example.

I have a zone on my soles between my toes and the arch where dead skin bubbles up and flakes off, similar to a blister but painless. Using a pumice stone every week to get rid of it in the shower keeps the skin loss to a minimum.

I've also noticed that my liner socks grip better because of that weekly ritual. Why is that a big deal? My liners can't rub and cause hot spots, which inevitably lead to blisters.

So make it a hiking habit to check out your feet, especially the bottoms. Then do a little preventive maintenance (fancy pedicures, optional).

7. **Avoid high heels in your non-trail life.**

The shoes you wear daily have a huge impact on how your hiking boots fit.

Are you a fan of heels? There are any number of reasons for avoiding high heels, including tight, sore muscles, back problems, and balance issues.

The link between high heels and blisters is this: Your feet become molded into the shape of your daily shoes much more so than your hiking boots, simply because of the amount of contact time and weight bearing in your daily routine.

When you plunge your foot into your hiking boot on your day off, after wearing heels for days on end, the contact points will be vastly different.

You will also be carrying more weight than usual on a hike, if you take the Ten Essentials (Chapter 2) advice to heart.

This sets you up for rubbed skin, and the creation of a blister (which is the separation of your epidermis from your underlying dermis, in case I didn't mention it earlier).

That's in addition to the muscle, back and balance problems mentioned above.

8. Hydrotherapy

Every chance you get on the trail, take off your boots and allow Mother Nature's cool waters, luscious mud and refreshing snow patches to caress your footsies!

Hiking hydrotherapy is a fast and easy way to connect with Mother Earth. And it gets the blood flowing out of the engorged blood vessels in your hard working feet in a jiffy!

No water around? At the very least, take off your boots and socks whenever possible. This allows air flow to dry out the damp skin between your toes.

While you're at it, wiggle those toes! Any kindness paid to your feet will be repaid a thousand fold on the trail.

FEMININE TRAIL HYGIENE

Now we get to the good stuff!

Hiking hygiene for women means dealing with (gasp!) **body fluids**.

Yuck, right?

Not so fast, dear hiker! Let's take a moment to *appreciate* those body fluids.

Then we can cover some hiking hygiene tips to keep your trail time hygienic as well as happy.

Hiking Hygiene for Women: SWEAT

SWEAT is the body's mechanism for safely dumping excess heat you generate during hiking. Chapter 4 explains this connection to hiking hydration.

Sweat (perspiration) doesn't start to smell until bacteria already living on your body (skin normal flora which fill up all of the cracks and crevices on your epidermis) go to work on it.

And consider this. If you didn't have sweat glands, you'd have to pant like a dog to keep your internal body temperature within a safe range during a hot hike. How unattractive would that be?

Drool on your pillow, not on the trail. That's what HFH always says :)

Sweating hard on a regular basis during exercise is great for flushing out toxins via the sweat. And it gets the lymphatic channels moving, too - important for a healthy immune system.

So do you REALLY want to wear an *anti*perspirant on the trail?

Instead, wear loose fitted hiking clothing with great ventilation and moisture wicking properties.

Tip: Tank tops, while a great way to keep your upper body cool, should have straps that are wide enough to cushion your skin from your backpack straps. Avoid tight clothing that doesn't wick away your sweat, because it will lead to painful chafing.

Don't forget to replace the water you lose in sweat. The more you sweat, the more you should be drinking water on the trail. Chapter 4 is all about hiking hydration.

More Juicy Body Fluids: URINE!

Urine is the way you let go of the substances your body doesn't need. So it's a good thing, right? Right!

Every time you urinate, you say good-bye to the end products of biochemical reactions your cells used to do work, as in:

-produce energy for your hike,

-keep your immune system strong,

-rebuild from injury or stress, and

-replenish themselves.

Urine comes from a sterile environment (your kidneys and bladder), so it's essentially "clean" in terms of microbial life. That's why you don't need to dig a hole before you pee.

Urine should not have an offensive odor. If it does, you might have a urinary tract infection. Keep on eye out for other symptoms:

-burning sensations during urination,

-fever and/or chills,

-dull ache in your upper back,

-along with cloudy, stinky urine.

These are symptoms you want to bring to a health care provider as soon as possible after your hike. In fact, turn around at the first signs of these problems and head home.

Do you know how to use the color and amount of your urine for immediate feedback about how hydrated you are (or aren't?) Read Chapter 4.

Allow me to give you some resources that can make this particular "hiking hygiene for women potential nightmare" [a.k.a."pit stop" or "pee break"] easier to handle.

Ready? Here we go...(really bad pun, sorry).

*Stand up when you pee, using a device designed to let you have the freedom of male anatomy. The upside? No squatting, and no need to pull down your drawers in less than ideal conditions: cold, wind, scratchy brush, rocky terrain with no handy coverage, to name just a few.

*Rather than trying to keep bulky toilet paper dry and clean, carry travel sized packs of disposable wipes in a hand made "hygiene kit", along with a plastic bag to receive the used ones. To call yourself a responsible hiker, pack out used wipes or toilet paper.

*Pick a pee spot way off the trail so wildlife isn't tempted to get ornery with passing hikers. Mountain goats, deer & chipmunks love to lick (and defend) the salts in your urine on rocks and logs.

*Forego the toilet paper and wipes altogether by using a pee rag! This idea is not for everyone. Guys are totally grossed out by it, which could be useful in certain situations.

Tip: Be sure the rag dries thoroughly in sunlight, and don't use it any other way. A dedicated rag ;)

OK, You Knew This Was Coming: BLOOD

Blood: the body's river of life, delivering oxygen to trillions of cells.

It carries away waste products, too, such as:

-carbon dioxide to the lungs for exhalation,

-toxic nitrogen compounds to the kidney for urination (see above),

-toxins in your food or medications, to be dealt with by the liver, and

-infectious organisms to the lymph nodes for destruction.

Hopefully, you're planning to keep your blood in your body (mosquitoes might steal a bit unless you're using the tips above on creepy crawly repellents).

But there's **monthly menstrual cycle blood** to think about if you're in a certain age bracket. Menstrual blood is definitely on the list as a hiking hygiene concern.

In fact, I know young women who stay off the trail during that time of the month. Don't let that be you!

This particular body fluid is released in relatively small amounts (compared with your total blood volume of 5 liters) when chemical messengers (hormones) tell the cells lining the uterus to slough off because there's no fertilized egg this month.

And away it goes, out of your body and into whatever receptacle you've chosen: tampon, sanitary napkin, or menstrual cup.

Tip: Menstrual blood should not have an offensive odor unless there's an infection in the reproductive tract. I am not saying it will be odorless, just that you shouldn't smell ammonia or other strong odors.

Your monthly cycle ties your body to the phases of the moon, to fertility, to your feelings about your body - and most importantly from a biology standpoint, this cycle guarantees the continuation of the human species.

All good reasons to honor the cycle, not dread it.

But realistically, you need to plan your hiking around your monthly flow. Don't avoid hiking, but be sure to carry the supplies you need, and pack out your used items. Hiking hygiene for women comes with the responsibility to make sure no one coming behind you on the trail knows that you've had to make that kind of pit stop.

Women sometimes wonder about the odor of menstrual blood attracting bears or other predators. Any truth to this worry about hiking hygiene for women?

The Journal of Wildlife Management published some research results in 1991 (a bit dated, but worthy of reading because bears today act pretty much like they did in 1991).

To bottom line it for you, NO - bears seem to prefer your food to your used "feminine hygiene" products. So go hiking, regardless of which day of the month it is! Just don't share your sandwich with a bear.

If you use paper products such as tampons and sanitary pads, be sure you've counted out, and packed, how many of these you'll be needing on your dayhike.

Then add a few extras, which can be used as fire starters or first aid supplies in emergencies.

Seal them in plastic bags, and double bag them because if they get wet or dirty, they're worthless.

Here's one approach to skipping the whole tampons/sanitary napkins supply issue: use an internal cup to catch your menstrual flow. The Diva Cup (see Chapter 6 Resources) gets high marks from female hikers.

There are a few precautions to note with a menstrual cup:

*Be sure your hands are *really, really clean* when you insert and remove it. Hand sanitizer is okay, but nothing beats soap and water for removing the most grime.

*Clean the cup and dispose of the menstrual fluids away from water sources or areas where other hikers might rest or camp.

Need some more tips on how to handle the "monthly issues" while on the trail, as well as other female hiker hygiene tips? Check the Resource section of this chapter.

Blood, Sweat... What's Next? *TEARS!*

If you're crying on the trail, chances are that you:

-are overcome with emotion at a spectacular waterfall,

-have just spotted a deceased (as in stinky) marmot *after you stepped on it,*

-have recently discovered a new species of stinging insect (congrats!),

-desperately need these tips for improving your trail techniques,

-or are suffering from blisters (see above).

Clearly, **hiking hygiene for women tips** are not uppermost on your mind.

Once you've recovered your equilibrium, rinse those sore eyes. They will feel so much better when you use the eye drops you included in your first aid kit.

See Chapter 6 Resources for details.

Oh, POOP. There's One More

Not to make light of the subject, but pooping in a cat hole is not that hard. But there are ways to make it even easier!

*Train your thigh muscles to squat. This makes you stronger on the trail, too.

*If squatting just isn't your thing, choose a poop spot that provides the luxury of leaning against a rock, hanging your bottom over a log, or some other way to relieve your thigh muscles of duty. Be aware that there are trade-offs to this (cold clammy rocks and splinters, to name a few).

*Use a lightweight trowel to prepare a cat hole before you get yourself lined up over it. Store this trowel in its own dedicated plastic bag.

*Baby wipes, paper towels, and hand sanitizer packed in a plastic bag will help you clean up. Don't neglect hand hygiene on the trail, especially if you share bags of trail snacks with your buddies.

*While urine is sterile, feces carries harmful microbes that should never enter water supplies. This includes tiny little trickles of streams, all the way up to the shorelines of big lakes. Be sure your cat hole is well away from water.

*If you have to resupply with surface water during your dayhike, don't trust that every other creature follows the rule above. Treat all water before consuming it, due to the possibility of viruses, bacteria and parasites carried in human and animal feces.

TRAIL ETIQUETTE

Now that you're fully prepared to be safe and comfortable on the trail, you need a few tips on trail etiquette to make you a safe, responsible member of the hiking community.

Just as in your social circles back home, there are ways to approach and interact with other hikers on the trail.

Who has the right of way on a narrow trail?

How do you yield safely to a horseback rider?

Rather than detail all of the answers for you, visit the Hiking For Her website for a free instant download pdf on Trail Etiquette which explains the rules of the trail, created by yours truly.

Now let's hike onward, to a brief look at trail ethics.

If you've heard the phrase "leave no trace", you'll find all the details about why that's important, coming right up.

LEAVE NO TRACE (LNT) PRINCIPLES

Leave No Trace hiking follows well established principles to keep your impact on the outdoors to a minimum.

Are there LNT police behind every tree, checking up on you?

No. But your own motivation to keep the outdoors free of tell tale signs of human activity will grow stronger with every day you spend beneath the open sky. It simply comes with the territory!

There are seven core principles in Leave No Trace hiking, all of them common sense and easy to practice.

Long story short: It's all about respect.

For the official version, visit the Leave No Trace Organization.

The abbreviated Hiking For Her version groups the principles into two big chunks of respect.

Anybody hearing Aretha Franklin right about now?

Respect for all life forms (yourself included)

-Plan ahead and prepare. (See Chapters 1-6)

-Respect wildlife's rhythms and habits. (Chapter 6).

-Be considerate of other visitors.

Respect for place

-Leave what you find. (Take photos before you leave.)

-Travel and take breaks on durable surfaces.

-Dispose of food and body wastes properly.

-Minimize campfire impacts if you have to stay overnight.

These Leave No Trace guiding principles aren't just for hikers.

Once you get hooked on this hiking thing, you'll find yourself applying them to your neighborhood park or any other outdoor space you visit.

And (hopefully) teaching them by words and deeds to the next generation on your dayhikes!

LNT Tips

Using these principles as guiding lights for your actions on a dayhike will become second nature to you (Mother Nature being your first love, right?).

Here are some tips for how to form good LNT habits as a hiker. Let's use the respectful approach again.

RESPECT FOR ALL LIFE FORMS, INCLUDING YOURSELF:

*Be meticulous in your planning.

-Do extensive online research about the permits you need, the terrain you'll be crossing, upcoming weather patterns, the mileage you'll be able to handle, trail conditions, adequate food and water intake, and trail regulations such as "no dogs".

-A prepared hiker stays found and safe while respecting the rules.

*Don't feed the bears, either accidentally or on purpose.

-If you're trekking through bear country, be bear aware and keep your lunch spot free of odors that might tempt a bear into bad behavior.

-A fed bear is a dead bear. Do you really want that on your conscience?

-Don't feed the squirrels, foxes, marmots or birds, either. They've survived without your help, and will need to do so after you walk away with your bag of delicious trail mix.

-Wildlife must respect the natural cycles in order to mate, reproduce and raise the next generation. So respect their rhythms and patterns.

*Keep your nose out of their business!

-Don't disturb their nests, dens and game trails.

-If you take photos, use a lens that allows you to keep your distance.

-If you find a "lost" baby animal, it probably isn't. Nature moms can't hire babysitters while they work to locate food.

*Hiking with dogs is as problematic as your dog is.

-I know, your dog is special, well trained and gentle as a lamb.

-But any dog gets crazy excited by the scent of deer or the dash of a squirrel across the trail.

-Know the regulations permitting or denying you the privilege of hiking with your dog, and respect why they are in place.

*On the trail, let this thought guide you to calm, quiet actions: Everyone is here for the same nature focused reasons.

-Voices on the trail can echo, bounce and amplify, so keep your conversations to low tones.

-Leave noise makers like ringing cells phones or music at home, or wear ear buds (not a recommended practice by HFH, for safety and enjoyment reasons, but it's an option for music and podcast lovers).

-Refrain from shouting your exuberance when you reach the top of the viewpoint. It disturbs life all around you. How about a victory dance instead?

*When you take a rest break on the trail, don't literally take it on the trail!

-Find a durable surface where you can sit, lounge, remove your boots, munch your peanuts, and dig through your pack without impeding the flow of other hikers.

-Leaving gouge marks and torn up plants once you get up? Just don't.

RESPECT FOR PLACE:

I feel somewhat sheepish about telling you to **leave what you find**, because I have been known to bring home bits of bone, goat hair, feathers, rocks and snail shells.

So I will take the high road and say that collecting freebies on the trail (mentioned above) is one thing, while digging up plants or destroying a rock face to snag a quartz crystal is quite another.

*Use durable surfaces for travel and campsites, especially in **fragile environments** such as alpine or desert terrains where plants struggle to gain, let alone maintain, a literal foot hold.

-Your feet may seem small in the vast outdoors, but to moss or lichen, they're immense and destructive.

*Being a biological entity generates **solid and liquid waste.**

-Use the tips for **hiking hygiene** in this chapter to start thinking about how to keep yourself and the environment clean as you release your blood, sweat, tears and feces into the environment.

*Humans also generate **waste during food preparation**.

-If you've done your planning (see the first principle) you've already minimized plastic or foil packaging.

-You have a "food loss prevention" plan in mind to deal with your wild neighbors.

-You bring only the amount you need.

-And you don't leave food behind to make trouble and unsightly messes for the next hikers to come along. Orange peels? Pack them out! Ditto for sunflower seed hulls.

*If you brought it in your pack, that's the way it leaves, too.

-No digging holes, no throwing it into the lake, no "hiding" it under a rock.

-That goes for paper, food scraps, and "garbage" such as used batteries or broken gear.

Leave No Trace Hiking summed up: a romantic, yet practical, ideal

If you've ever yearned to melt into the landscape without a trace, living by your wits (and the technology in your pack) while glimpsing wildlife and marinating in awe inducing vistas, you're my kinda hiker!

Apply the LNT principles to make sure I can't trace you.

And rest assured that I'm returning the favor.

Because fossilized orange peels and brown toilet paper aren't what I want to see on the trail.

And I'm not interested in seeing your initials on the tree outside my tent.

Or finding your dirty socks at the lake I worked hard to reach.

I'm sure that you and I agree on the wisdom of Leave No Trace hiking principles. Glad you're on the trail with me, Leave No Trace Hiking virtual trail buddy!

Chapter 6 Summed Up

This chapter was a long one, wasn't it!

That's because there are so many things you can do to keep yourself safe and comfortable during a day hike.

Which of the suggestions in this chapter resonated most deeply with you?

And which ones did you shy away from?

Those are your strengths and deficits.

Now it's up to you to shore up your deficits, and keep adding to your strengths.

Don't forget that you can contact me via the HFH website with your questions and suggestions!

Chapter 6 Take Aways

Hike your own hike. That means look after your own comfort and safety, and go at your own pace.

If you **feel creeped out by someone** at the trailhead or on the trail, don't bury that feeling. **Take action** to remove yourself pronto.

Expect (and respect) animal, bird and insect encounters.

Bookmark the free U.S. government NOAA site for North America, and make it a habit to consult it for **weather conditions** before each hike.

Use your ten essentials if an emergency or injury occurs. Keep a **calm, focused attitude** and **choose the best option** for rescue.

Your feet are an important asset on a hike. **Blister prevention** means paying attention to hot spots and responding immediately.

Blood, sweat, urine, tears and poop are part of the trail experience. Don't let them keep you off from hiking.

Trail etiquette is an unwritten code of honor to respect other people on the trail.

Leave No Trace principles extend that respect to all that surrounds you.

Chapter Six Resources

Hiking For Her Recommendations and Additional Information for Safety and Comfort

READING THE WEATHER

In order to understand what the weather is up to, you'll have to learn a bit about meteorology(the study of the ocean of air surrounding Earth). Here's a painless way to do it.

A fabulous company called The Teaching Company identifies the best college professors, and records them giving lectures.

Their Meteorology series has 24 lectures in all, 30 minutes each. There's a booklet which summarizes the main points of each lecture, too.

You can watch them whenever you have the time or inclination. (FYI: I have no affiliate connection to them, I just love their products. They run frequent sales, too.)

The 30 minute segments present basic physics concepts (temperature, pressure, density), take a look at the layers of atmosphere, and talk about radiation & the greenhouse effect. And that's just the beginning.

If this sounds too detailed for you, try a few books by Richard Hamblyn. Seems he's a bit of a weather geek.

My current favorite gives an incredible amount of information packed into a small space, and you gotta love the title, right? The Cloud Book.

I must admit, I never realized how many types of clouds there are. How often do you pay attention to the sky when you hike? (After reading this chapter, you should say "a lot").

And who knew they had elaborate names such as "altocumulus stratiformis" and (even better) "cirrus spissatus cumulonimbogenitus".

I kid you not.

The dramatic color photos alone are worth the price of the book. Tormenting your friends & neighbors with those absurdly long words: optional fun.

The Hiking For Her website has many articles related to weather safety. Use these keywords to find them:

-Lightning Safety

-Hiking Weather

-Rain Gear

TRAIL STRESS

Here's a preventative approach to trail stress: Do some reading about extreme situations before you get caught in one.

Many fatalities could have been prevented by avoiding panicked decisions.

Knowing how to survive unpleasant outdoor situations prevents those panicked decisions, and saves lives - yours, in this case.

Visit the HFH website for articles on solo hiking stress. These tips can be applied to group hiking as well.

BLISTERS

To prevent hot spots from forming on your toes, and thus preventing blisters, try high performance socks (Chapter 1).

Here's an alternative to duct tape: Leukotape. It breathes better but the stickiness rapidly disappears if trail grit gets on it or your fingers touch it too much. Practice at home first. And use the scissors from your first aid kit to cut it to fit.

One more duct tape alternative: a very thin bandage with a "bubble" to keep heat and friction from wreaking havoc on your skin: Blisto-O-Ban Medical Adhesive.

Oops! Got a blister anyway?

Blister treatment is pretty straightforward, but you need to pack a few supplies.

Try this magic stuff! I carry it in my pack "just in case": Glacier Gel Blister and Burn Dressing.

Moleskin is a famous, and reliable, way to keep a blister contained. It's easily obtained in any pharmacy.

And now for the fun part: Deciding if you're a blister popper, or not. Read the HFH article on blisters to help you decide when you should, and when you shouldn't pop these bad boys.

INFLAMMATION

These are the products I use routinely to fight muscle inflammation after a long hike: Tiger Balm and Mineral Ice.

With either of these products, **WASH YOUR HANDS before touching your eyes or mouth,** or you'll be sorry! You'll have inflamed eyes to go along with the rest of your hiking inflammation.

By relieving the muscle soreness with these topical approaches, you are helping flush the muscles of lactic acid and other compounds produced during exercise.

That's going to reduce the healing time between hikes, especially if coupled with proper hydration and good nutrients.

Yet another topical approach to combating soreness and inflammation: Topricin cream.

A nice long **soak in a hot bathtub saturated with Epsom salts (magnesium sulfate)** is the cheapest way to buy relief from muscle pain and stiffness after a hike. Epsom salts are easy to find in local drug stores and some grocery stores.

If you're not a "bath" type of person, soak a soft cloth in Epsom-saturated warm water and apply it to your sore areas.

This works for reversing hiking inflammation, trust me! You will feel SO much better after this old fashioned, low tech, cheap combination of minerals and hydrotherapy.

CHAFING

To deal with chafing issues *anywhere* on your body, try this "slippery on purpose" product: Body Glide. There are various formulations, some made specifically for women.

Or try a product called Bag Balm. Weird name, but it has a good track record with hikers dealing with chafed skin.

Tip: In a pinch, use your lip balm to lubricate the affected areas.

INSECT REPELLENTS

Sometimes your clothing is the best repellent. Long sleeves, long pants, neck gaiters, hats... read Chapter 1 for some tips.

If you opt for full strength DEET, use it sparingly, because it's heavy duty stuff.

I've had good success with herbal insect repellents in buggy terrain.

Up to a point.

Which is why a bug net is a perfect back up plan.

Full disclosure: No repellent works 100% of the time.

Try an "after bite" product to minimize the discomfort of insect bites. I've had good success with it on my own mosquito and fly bites.

And this counts as an extra kindness when hiking with children.

FEMININE HYGIENE TRAIL PRODUCTS

Stand up if you're ready to pee like the guys!

Here are 2 popular choices for "female urination devices": Go Girl and SheWee (clever names or what?).

Pre-moistened wipes are a great idea for cleaning up. Travel packs are your best option.

For handling menstrual flow, use a Diva Cup menstrual cup. But be sure you use the right size. Look at the marketing information and select the one that fits your situation.

For a lengthy discussion of female hiker hygiene concerns, visit these articles on the HFH website:

Hiking Hygiene For Women

Best Female Hiker Hygiene Tips: How To Stay Clean On The Trail

EYE CARE

Adding lubricating drops to my eyes doesn't sting, and soothe my irritated eyeballs quickly so I can get back to hiking, or resting.

I predict that you'll be grossed out by the amount of trail dirt floating around on your eyeballs and lids.

Choose a brand with no chemicals or preservatives.

Just a reminder: Polarized sunglasses are one of the ten essentials. See Chapter 2 Resources for suggestions.

Hiking For Her Additional Information

INFLAMMATION

Harvard Health Publications offers tips in this article: Foods That Fight Inflammation

ANIMAL ENCOUNTERS

If you don't know bear safety practices, read them at http://dnr.alaska.gov/parks/safety/bear

Cougar safety tips: www.env.gov.bc.ca/wld/documents/cougsf.htm

TRAIL ETIQUETTE

American Hiking Society offers standard trail etiquette tips.

Seattle Backpackers Magazine has even more trail etiquette tips.

LNT PRINCIPLES

Applying Leave No Trace hiking principles are the only way to feel good about yourself as a strong female hiker. They bring new meaning to the phrase "pay it forward". Read the complete HFH article for more the details, as well as the Socially Responsible Hiking article.

Chapter 7: Navigation and Communication

Getting lost might lead to five minutes of fame on the evening news, but it's not a recommended hiking strategy for a dayhiker.

Want to avoid being interviewed as you limp out of the woods in mud smeared clothes at midnight? Here are the things you need to know to stay out of the lost and found category:

-Three ways to use a hiking map

-The value of hiking pedometers

-GPS as a navigation tool

-When to rely on cell phone coverage

-The difference between a personal locator beacon and a satellite messenger

As always, let's jump right in.

HIKING NAVIGATION AND COMMUNICATION

Hiking women today have access to a staggering variety of hiking navigation aids, including

-satellite-detailed maps,

-Google Earth (free download, with hiking trails marked in bright red),

-World Wind from NASA,

-global positioning systems (GPS),

-personal locator devices,

-satellite messengers.

And when all else fails, you could fall back on time tested methods of dead reckoning to find your route.

Regardless of which navigation system you use, the underlying fundamental is knowledge. This same idea came up in Chapter 6, didn't it!

Acquiring knowledge will cost you some time and effort to figure out which navigational tools are the most important for the type of hiking you do. But don't begrudge that time investment, along with the money you invest in it.

Staying found (as in, not getting lost) means that you don't inconvenience, scare, or endanger other people.

Sounds like a worthy goal, wouldn't you agree?

Tip: Be sure to count yourself in on that worthy goal! Peace of mind as a hiker is worth way more than the money it takes to ensure that you can navigate safely in all weather conditions.

Let's start with ways to use those maps you acquired in Chapter 5.

THREE WAYS TO USE HIKING MAPS

There are at least three fun ways to use maps. Folding them into impromptu party hats does not count, even though that sounds like fun.

If you cringe at the sight of "fun" and "maps" in the same sentence, you probably skipped Chapter 5.

Please read it now, to learn the details of **using a map for planning a hike**, including locating the right access roads, finding the trailhead, picking the best hiking destination, and establishing a turn around time.

Already on board with how useful maps are for planning a hike?

Great! Here's **the second way** to use a map: **to estimate mileage for pacing**.

This might not sound like something you would like to do, at first glance. But it's a useful skill once you've been on enough dayhikes to get a feel for how ambitious your hiking plans should be for a given set of circumstances.

Chapter 8 gives you all the details on hiking pacing. For now, let's consider this example of how maps and pacing are intertwined.

One day you decide that your next hike will be to Lake Serenity. You whip out your topographical map (the one with contour lines indicating elevation gain and loss) and you see that your hike starts at 1200 feet.

Your objective, Lake Serenity, lies at 3400 feet above sea level.

Knowing that you need to gain 3400 – 1200 = 2200 feet to arrive at your destination, and knowing how many miles it takes to reach the lake, you can calculate how fast you need to move.

Two miles per hour might be just right, but for a rainy day on a slick trail it might be too ambitious. And it is an uphill hike, so even on a fair weather day you should dial back your estimated pace. That means you'll have to leave the trailhead a bit earlier.

See how you can fine-tune your hiking plans? That gives you control over your hiking destiny.

And by building up a mental repertoire of "what if" scenarios, you can select the right hike in unknown terrain, and get it right just about every time.

Your trail buddies will admire this. Heck, you will admire this about yourself!

Bottom line: You want to cultivate the knack of being realistic about how long it will take to achieve your hiking objective(s) AND get yourself back to the trailhead with plenty of daylight to spare.

Maps can definitely get you there (a shameless map pun).

Here's **a third way to use hiking maps**: to **scout interesting land features and topography** that you can explore during the hike.

Interesting is in the eye of the beholder, but a few examples include high points for unimpeded vistas, hidden lakes, potential waterfall areas, old mines, logging roads to ridges for viewpoints, swampy areas for botanical specimens – all of these provide an open door for adventures!

If you're the type of dayhiker who prefers to have a little solitude, scope out your possibilities on the map.

For instance, large easy-to-reach lakes (as in popular destinations for noisy families) might be right on the trail, but perhaps there's a small (quiet, peaceful) lake just a little ways off the trail that you could visit - if you knew the coordinates. The map knows all.

And wouldn't it be cool to know ahead of time where you could climb a hill to get a better view and snap some photos that no one else can get?

HIKING PEDOMETERS

Now that you know how many miles you're going to cover, why not verify it with a pedometer? This is literally a meter for measuring feet, or footsteps in this case.

There's a good reason why I recommend using one. Checking your pedometer at regular intervals gives you a sense of **what mileage feels like**.

You can use this kinesthetic "feel" for mileage to estimate how far you've gone at any particular point during a hike – and then check it on the device. Very useful for pacing!

And with a pedometer, you can **quantify your body's reaction** to your hike. Examples: You will notice what one mile feels like on various terrains, how your knee starts acting up around five miles, and when you've hit double digit mileage because your toes start to cramp.

Once you have enough practice at this, when you meet someone on the trail who asks you "How much farther to the lake?" you can give them an amazingly reliable estimate without consulting the map.

Tracking mileage also makes the symbols on a piece of paper (i.e. a hiking map) come alive in a new dimension.

A pedometer is not a hiking essential, but it can be fun to wear one. Chapter 7 Resources will point you toward the good ones.

NAVIGATION AND COMMUNICATION

A dayhiker who sticks to a well marked trail is navigating in a low tech, reliable manner.

Until there comes an inevitable day when the trail signs have been used for target practice. Or they are missing altogether at a confusing intersection where you need them the most.

Then the question becomes "Where am I?"

Followed quickly by "What's my next move?"

There are several ways to get the answers to your questions. Let's look at each of them in turn:

-Global Positioning System (GPS)

-Cell phones

-Personal Locator Beacons (PLB)

-Satellite messengers

GPS NAVIGATION

GPS (Global Positioning System) as a navigational tool is not something every dayhiker needs to invest in. Nothing beats the low cost and reliability of a map and compass.

In fact, GPS is a dying technology that is being replaced by everyone's access to cell phones and portable devices for satellite communications.

For these reasons, Hiking For Her is not a big fan of GPS for dayhikers, but in an effort to give you an idea of what using one might be like, here are a few facts.

-GPS navigation needs a clear view of the sky, because it must acquire signals from multiple satellites orbiting the Earth.

So if you hike in dense forests or in deep canyons, you won't be able to use it to pinpoint your location reliably.

Thick cloud cover might also screw up a signal, leaving you wondering where the heck you are.

-In addition, the user interface on most GPS units is fiddly and requires an investment of time to learn how to operate.

Some have fairly steep learning curves.

-GPS relies on batteries, so if you're not diligent about battery maintenance you'll be out of luck. Battery life is decreased in cold conditions, something to keep an eye on during winter hikes or at high elevation.

CELL PHONES

Cell phones are becoming commonplace in our increasingly connected world.

There are several issues of concern to consider if you are going to rely exclusively on your cell phone to navigate while hiking (as well as to communicate with the off trail world in an emergency).

Signal coverage is one problem that you probably thought of first. No signal, no navigating. Also, no sending or receiving messages. The more remote or mountainous your day hike, the more likely you are without service.

And there's no way to know ahead of time whether or not you'll have cell phone coverage. You might want to take notes during your favorite hikes of where coverage was spotty or non-existent, and carry alternate navigational tools on hikes in those areas.

Battery life is another problem. If your phone requires daily charging, and you are using it heavily to check your location and to send text messages, take photos, make notes (as above), or update your social media accounts – well, you know the rest of that sad story.

On the other hand, there are some dandy map and navigational apps for your phone (see Resources at the end of the chapter). With prudent usage, in the right location, a charged cell phone is invaluable for figuring out where you are.

Some apps allow you to record your entire hike: distance, elevation gain and loss, time spent moving, and more. This makes a fun way to share your hike with others who ask what your favorite hikes are.

But don't pin all your hopes on a cell phone's ability to keep you found. It could turn out to be the weakest link in your hiking plan.

PERSONAL LOCATORS

Personal locator beacons do pretty much what they promise: **locate your person, and report your position** to someone who will perform a "search and rescue" for you.

You have to be in a **dire emergency situation** to consider activating it.

-A broken trekking pole doesn't count.

-Spotting a bear two ridges over doesn't count.

-A medical emergency that would be labeled a 911 situation at home, *now you're talking*.

Except that you won't be talking.

Unlike your cell phone, there is no two-way communication available with these beacons. A PLB is designed for one thing: to send an *emergency* message for help.

It's important to understand and accept those distinctions, because once you hit the "HELP" button, your message goes to some pretty high powered folks:

-National Oceanic and Atmospheric Administration: NOAA,

-Air Force Rescue Coordination Center: AFRCC,

-Search and Rescue Satellite Aided Tracking: an international cooperation of military satellites with the acronym COSPAS-SARSAT.

They won't be pleased to rescue someone with a broken trekking pole, if you take my meaning.

And to rub salt into the wound, the cost of your rescue, regardless of how "legitimate" it is, gets billed to YOU.

So if you plan on carrying a personal locator beacon, be very sure you need to deploy it before sending that emergency message. Because these babies work, and work very well, to send an SOS that will get you rescued ASAP (oops, fell into the acronym trap again).

There are some realities about a PLB that should be crystal clear before you purchase one for dayhiking. To make it short and simple:

-You must register your PLB device with NOAA to receive a unique identifying number, which will be used when locating you. Registration is free, but if you forget to do it, your device is useless in an emergency situation.

-These devices use satellites, so you must be in a position where the device and the satellites can "see" each other (just like GPS, covered above). Deep canyons, thick forests, sometimes even dense clouds or blocking the signal with your pack dumps you into the SOL category (darn it! I'm trying to break free!).

-If your signal is transmitted at night, you will have to wait until daylight plus clear weather for a helicopter or land based rescue team to arrive. Ten Essentials (Chapter 2) to the rescue while you wait for the rescue!

-The accuracy of your locator signal depends on which type of PBL you buy. If it uses GPS (the recommended, and more expensive, option), you'll be assured of rescuers pinpointing you to within 100 meters in 5 minutes or less. That's impressive!

-Without a GPS interface, accuracy drops to 2 miles before switching to a different frequency to pinpoint you more exactly. Why does this matter? Time. If you're bleeding or losing consciousness, time is of the essence.

-This is a battery-dependent device, so it's only as reliable as your commitment to perform regular battery checks/replacement. Also, cold temperatures will eat into the battery life. These were also concerns with the GPS unit, right?

-You must flip the "on" switch to activate the signal transmission. It doesn't transmit continuously, which makes sense, given the SOS nature of its signal. But if you're physically unable to throw the switch, the device is useless.

Do you need to carry a personal locator beacon?

Only you can answer this question.

Dayhikers take less risks than backpackers, because they rack up less trail time. Yet hiking remains an unpredictable sport for all hikers.

Dayhikers who do moderate length hikes on clearly marked trails, and make a point to use the trail best practices outlined in this book, have a low (but never zero) rate of getting into emergency situations.

So if you don't take many risks, always stay within easy reach of civilization, and have documented beforehand that you can rely on cell phone coverage on your hike, you probably don't need to carry a PLB.

But if you risk going into the backcountry, especially in extreme weather conditions through isolated regions, or hike rugged terrain (river crossings, predator encounters, steep unstable footing), *and you do so regularly*, perhaps it's time to take a look at these devices.

Calculate for yourself the worth of what you are purchasing:

-Lightweight peace of mind when taking risks away from civilization,

-Free registration,

-Assurance of rescue where ever you wander (with weather and daylight constraints).

But don't forget:

-You bear the full cost of the rescue (helicopters aren't cheap!).

-A PLB is not a trivial piece of hiking gear to purchase; average cost hovers around $300.

-Battery maintenance is your responsibility.

-Emergencies only! Define EMERGENCY as life threatening issues requiring immediate attention.

-There is no two-way transmission; only a "HELP" message will be sent (and may not be sent and/or received, depending on where you are).

-Get out from under trees, into as much open space with a view of the sky as possible, before you activate your PLB. Give the signal the best chance of finding its target satellites.

-Once the message is sent, the genie is out of the bottle, so to speak. You can't take it back!

Just to reiterate: If you're a casual dayhiker on established trails, you probably don't need a device of this technological sophistication.

But if you hike alone frequently (your canine companion doesn't count), or venture off established trails, you should consider the merits of a lightweight portable personal locator beacon.

One more tip: If you activate your PLB, do everything you can to make yourself highly visible to the rescuers. Some PLBs have LED strobe lights to assist with this.

If you carry a reflective space blanket, a whistle, a shiny old CD or DVD, use all of those to attract attention once you hear the helicopter or see rescuers approaching.

And if you do buy a PLB, be your own best friend and register it immediately.

Then add "battery checks" to your hiking calendar.

If you rely upon your hiking buddy to carry it, don't feel weird about asking if these things have been done. This falls into the "Better safe than sorry" category of trail etiquette.

Not convinced that a PLB sounds right for you? Maybe you need to carry a **SEND** device instead (Satellite Emergency Notification Device).

SATELLITE MESSENGERS

Satellite messengers for hikers at first glance seem like a no brainer. Who wouldn't want to carry a communication device that can help you out of a jam?

But wait! Isn't that your cell phone?

As already discussed, the pivotal question becomes "Will your cell phone coverage be reliable where you're going, and exactly when you need it?" (see above)

Enter **satellite messengers**: more than just a hand held device for sending an SOS message to initiate rescue from nasty circumstances (like a PLB) or a cell phone (to phone home).

The benefits of light weight emergency satellite messenger devices for hikers include:

-One-way message sending, or two-way messaging (for a higher price point). These are non-emergency messages, so you can pinpoint your location for loved ones at home, but also update them and answer questions.

-The device can track you, making you visible to folks interested in your hiking progress in real time.

-It can also send an SOS message.

-The battery life is reasonably long, although cold conditions will cut into battery performance.

Satellite messengers make sense when you are doing a hike that loved ones are not completely on board with. One example: a solo female hiker who is navigating unfamiliar trails or going into the backcountry, with anxious loved ones biting their nails back home.

Now for the drawbacks:

-These devices are not cheap. Only you can decide if the investment makes sense for your style of hiking.

-You have to pay to play. In other words, add a subscription fee to your hiking budget. If you're a frequent hiker, a yearly fee makes sense. If you're not, choose a company that charges a monthly fee that can be canceled without penalty, or offers a reasonable data plan to fit your trail time.

-Time lags between "send" and "receive" may occur, weakening the effectiveness of the messages.

-Messages may not send, depending on your ability to access the satellites and the strength of the signal. This creates stress in the people expecting an "all okay" message - the exact opposite of your intent. It could also give you a false sense of hope.

-An unobstructed view of the sky is necessary before trying to send or receive a message. If you hike in areas where this isn't possible, the device will be dead weight in your pack.

-These messengers can be hard/clunky to use, with variable size and weight. This cuts down their effectiveness for less-than-dedicated users.

To sum it up, you're going to have to do some careful research before purchasing one of these gizmos, because not every one does every thing listed above.

Decide what's most important to you, and then buy the device that excels in those things: messages, tracking, rescue or all three.

Decision time for navigation technology: to buy or not to buy

You have to ask yourself some questions before you can decide which piece of navigational technology works best for your style of hiking.

-Do you want to be able to send and receive messages while hiking?

-If so, will your cell phone be reliable?

-Do you want to make yourself "trackable" during your hike?

-Are you going into areas where an SOS rescue is more than a faint possibility?

-Do you hike in areas that are hard to access and might require a helicopter evacuation?

-How much is the "luxury" of communication worth to you? Not only in terms of money, but in terms of weight, ease of use, reliability and peace of mind?

These are questions only you can answer!

If all you want is a panic button for an emergency rescue, consider carrying a PLB.

But if you want it all (communication, tracking, AND rescue messaging), satellite messengers are here for you.

If you didn't catch my hesitation to rely on cell phones while hiking, here it is in one blatant sentence: **Carry a cell phone, but rely on it only in the best of circumstances.**

Chapter 7 Summed Up

It's great to know where you're going. Maps are a splendid invention that give you a bird's eye view of your hike.

And there are several ways to use them, as you just found out.

If you find yourself "navigationally challenged" (ahem!) in your daily life, pay particular attention to this chapter.

You know who you are: can't find your car in the parking lot, get turned around in a shopping mall, have no idea which way is north.

No shame in all that, but don't let it lead you down the wrong trail during a hike. It's a deficit that can be fixed with learning to read maps. And technology.

So here's a not-so-fun assignment: spend some time imagining what you would do if you lost the trail, or lost your balance and took a tumble on the trail. How would you get rescued? This chapter laid out your options.

Now it's up to you to decide which piece of technology suits you best.

Chapter 7 Take-Aways

Form a map addiction early in your career as a hiker.

Plan your hike with maps and carry them in your pack regardless of how "easy" or short the hike seems.

A **hiking pedometer enhances your awareness** of the trail.

Technology can be an aid, but will cost you time and money.

Devices that rely on **satellite signals** require an unobstructed view of the sky.

Don't rely on **cell phone coverage** during your hike.

A **charged battery is priceless** on the trail, regardless of which device it powers. Always leave home with fully charged batteries.

Chapter 7 Resources

Hiking For Her Navigation Recommendations

Pedometers

If you want to multi-task, see if you can use an app on your cell phone to count your daily activity level. I use one called **Calorie Counter & Diet Tracker by MyFitnessPal.com**.

There is a entire universe of pedometers. Tip: Be sure to read all of the reviews, and use the "compare" features to zero in on the pedometer of your dreams.

Personal Locator Beacons

Alright, time to do some serious thinking about whether or not you need a way to transmit a one-way SOS message for immediate rescue from a trail emergency.

I don't carry one myself, although I have been on hiking trips where PLBs were carried.

Here's one that gets good reviews: ACR Electronics RESQLink + GPS personal locator beacon. Recall that the GPS feature makes the rescue process go faster, and thus is worth the additional cost.

Satellite Communicators

I read reviews all the time, and based on what I've read, I can recommend this device: DeLorme InReach SE Two-Way Satellite Communicator.

Here's why:

-It's easy to use. That's worth it's weight in gold, because if you are befuddled by the buttons, or have to remember a lot of technical details each time you turn it on, you're not going to use it (correctly).

-Reliability is high, given the field testing done with it. You don't want to be hiking along, thinking that your messages have been sent, when they have not left the device.

-At the time of this writing, there is no annual activation fee, meaning you can customize your usage.

-It uses the top satellite network available (2016), called Iridium.

-With batteries, weight comes in under one pound.

-If you want more features, the DeLorme InReach Satellite Explorer model will deliver them. The price point will be higher, so be sure you can justify those features.

Hiking For Her Additional Information

Stanford Medicine News Center has an interesting article on how pedometers help you stay active.

tchester.org/znet/grand_canyon/pedometer_accuracy.html asks, and answers, the question: How accurate are pedometers?

Chapter 8: Pacing

Best trail advice on pacing: Start off slow and cool, and then use your body's clues to tackle the changing terrain and weather.

Okay, we're done!

Not so fast. Here's what you'll discover about those clues in Chapter 8:

-The Number One Pacing Rule for women hikers

-How to find the best hiking pace

-Stride and pole adjustments for changing terrain and mileage

-The "Soaked Shirt" rule for female hikers

Pacing is fun, you'll see!

NUMBER ONE HIKING PACING RULE

As hikers, let's not beat around any bushes. Here's the most important pacing rule:

Always hike your own hike.

You've probably heard this little gem of trail wisdom before. Long trail hikers spout this platitude to mean that if you're not hurting anyone else, anything goes on a thru hike.

But what does it mean *for you*?

Well, for starters, it means that sometimes you have to let go of your preconceived ideas about how your hike "should" go.

It also means that you can't give in to group pressures that decide how fast, far or hard to hike on any particular dayhike.

Here's a likely scenario that can trigger anxiety while trying to hike your own hike.

Your trail buddies are going too fast for comfort but you are reluctant to say anything. In your head, there could be many issues that hold you back from speaking up:

-Subtle, or overt, competition,

-Expectations about gender or age behaviors,

-Performance pressure,

-Self doubt,

-Physical limitations or injuries that you don't want to reveal.

Any or all of these unspoken issues keep you from speaking your truth, which leads to hating the hike, and maybe never hiking with those folks again.

If you feel any shame or embarrassment about being "the slow hiker" or "the contrarian", you're not going to enjoy your trail time.

So here's the punch line of "hiking your own hike":

Don't ALLOW anyone, male or female, young or old, to take away your power as a female hiker.

Need some strategies to keeping your power on the trail? I just happen to have a few handy.

STRATEGIES FOR POWER FILLED HIKING

Idea #1: *FIND YOUR PERSONAL COMFORT ZONE*

Here's how to do this.

Plan a half-day hike near your home. On the hike, go as slow or fast as you'd like. Give yourself permission to adjust your pace according to your mood or curiosity.

Allow trail conditions to give you feedback about your pace: breathing rate, leg strength, muscle twinges, amount of sweat. Receive the feedback without judgment (too fast, too weak, etc.).

Chapter 7 outlines how to use a hiking pedometer to develop a feel for pacing yourself. This might be a nice gift to yourself.

Bring something unusual and delicious for lunch, trail food that you really look forward to eating.

And pack a camera, sketch pad, field guide, book of poems, or whatever says "fun" to you. Stop when the mood strikes and *enjoy yourself*! There is absolutely no pressure to achieve, conquer, or perform.

If you'd like, experiment with pushing yourself a little bit, or backing off even though your head tells you "should" go faster. Can you find your best trail rhythm?

You'll know you've come into your power when you feel strong, confident and energetic. You won't be able to keep a happy hiker smile off your face!

What you've done is find **your personal comfort zone**, without anyone but yourself giving you feedback about how fast/slow you "should" be going.

And most importantly, you are giving yourself permission to enjoy your hike. Isn't that the entire point?

Idea #2: **USE A DOG PACE**

Borrow a dog to hike with, or invite yours along on your next dayhike.

It goes without saying that it's a well behaved, leash trained animal that you have good verbal rapport with (the dog listens to voice commands related to the trail).

Check ahead of time to know that you're on a trail that welcomes canines. Some areas require that you use a leash, others don't allow dogs. Leave No Trace principles (Chapter 7) are why you need to respect those rules.

As the two of you hike along, watch how the dog enjoys simply moving through space, fully inhabiting its body as it adjusts to the trail conditions.

Sometimes the dog goes faster, sometimes more slowly in order to savor a particularly juicy trail offering.

The dog is hiking its own hike, right there beside you! Dog as mentor, it's a beautiful thing.

Another thing to note: when it's time to rest, the dog relaxes into the moment and doesn't feel bad about feeling tired. When you call a halt, why not do the same?

Idea #3: **WOMEN ONLY**

Join, or start, a woman's hiking group in your area. Zero in on the age range and level of ambition that resonates with your idea of a good time on the trail.

I've had success with putting up signs in coffee shops and bookstores. You could also try MeetUp groups for your area.

Tip: Be very clear about what type(s) of hiking companions you are looking to find. If you've been burned in the past, specify "no hard cores". (They pride themselves on the label, and can be a pain to hike with if your pace doesn't match theirs. I mean that quite literally.)

Idea #4: **LIGHTEN UP**

If you really want to go faster and expend less effort on the trail, examine your gear. Where could your dump some weight?

See Chapter 8 Resources for some ideas.

Idea #5: **SET BOUNDARIES**

Remind yourself that you have every right to hike the hike that's right for you, not an imposed idea of the perfect hike.

Then practice speaking up for yourself on the trail. Hear yourself say "I need to slow things down a little."

If you're not ready to swim against the group current, how does a trial run of speaking up in front of the mirror make you feel?

-Practice until you believe that you deserve to hike your own hike.

-If you're in the right hiking circles, people will understand and be receptive to your needs.

-Otherwise, find different trail buddies.

HIKING PACE

Some people are "*fast starters*" in terms of hiking pace. They practically run up the trail, before their muscles have had a chance to get warmed up.

They remain oblivious to their cold muscles, or are determined to "get a head start" - as if the hike is a race.

Other people are "*slow starters*". They hike for ten minutes, then stop to make multiple adjustments to gear, or look for a snack, or consult the map, or just want to talk about the weather.

Somehow they are resistant to getting warmed up and rolling along at a steady pace. Or maybe they forgot to calculate a turn around time? (Chapter 5)

While there's nothing wrong with making adjustments and being attuned to your comfort level, it's going to be tough for muscles to get into the proper rhythm at an inconsistent hiking pace. This is especially true when you first start down the trail.

Why not try for the middle ground: "*not too fast, not too slow*".

After you go through your trailhead routine (Chapter 6), start off at a *slow, reasonable hiking pace* for at least ten minutes.

Then ramp up (or down) from there to your *optimal speed*, given the terrain, weather conditions, and how your legs are feeling that day.

Check in with yourself and pay attention to how you're feeling after about 30 minutes of hiking. Then use that data to fine tune your hiking pace to external and internal factors that affect your hiking pace.

Sounds like a lot of self awareness, doesn't it? But it pays off in a more enjoyable hike.

Tip: Don't beat yourself up because your last hike (especially if it was on the same trail) felt effortless compared to the current one! Every day is a new day on the trail.

Many Factors Affect Hiking Pace

Ever have one of those days when your legs feel like cement? Or your lungs are burning after just 5 minutes of uphill work? You probably wonder what the heck is going on!

Learn to give in gracefully on those days, and slow your pace. If you try to ignore the feedback signals and forge ahead at a too-fast pace, your body will pay you back later by not wanting to reach the summit, or being sore the next day.

And on days when your legs feel great? Smile a great big hiker smile, pick up the pace until you "hit the wall"*, then back off slightly and maintain that pace.

*Note: Hitting the wall can mean many things, including ragged tortured breathing, a "stitch" in your side, lots of sweat suddenly pouring down your back and neck, along with burning thigh & leg muscles.

Every fiber of your hiking being says STOP, or at least SLOW DOWN. You won't be able to ignore these signals.

Know that your menstrual and sleep cycles, along with recent eating and hydration patterns, will also influence your hiking pace more than you would like to admit.

Another factor that can affect your pace? Unavoidable trail conditions.

It's not possible to know ahead of time if there are downed tree limbs or deep ruts left by dirt bikes or piles of horse poop on the trail (unless you were lucky enough to hear it through the grape vine or read a current trail report).

What if it rained the night before, leaving deep mud holes to negotiate? That will definitely slow you down, unless your gaiters and boots (Chapter 1) are up to the task of plowing through the muck.

There's also the possibility that a stretch of trail is closed or re-routed for maintenance. Or maybe animal activity such as elk breeding season or grizzly sightings forced a temporary trail closure.

Be philosophical about all of these possibilities. If you have to go slower, so be it.

Of course, it will eat into your turn-around time (see Chapter 5), but perhaps you can make up the time higher up or farther along the trail. Again, your topographical maps will give you this information.

Check the map for an alternate destination, too. Sometimes you might have to "settle" for a less spectacular objective, but at least you're hiking, right?

As you deal with the trail impediments, keep a running mental tab on how much time remains until you reach your turn around time so that you don't get into a time bind.

You could also set a timer on your watch or phone, and when it's turn around time, guess what you should do? Turn around!

And there's one big pacing impediment which is non-negotiable: meeting a bear on the trail. Don't even think twice. Backtrack or deviate, and allow the bear at least 30 minutes to clear out before venturing back onto the trail. You're in his/her big back yard, after all!

Tip: Be extra cautious if you spot adorable bear cubs. You know the stories about mama bear's bad manners, and they're all true. Same goes for mama moose, mother mountain goats and mommy marmots.

Okay, probably not marmots.

The terrain dictates pace, too. Knowing the terrain before hand, to whatever extent is possible, allows you to calculate the pace needed to reach your objective by the turn-around time (Chapter 5).

It also allows you to set the proper mental expectations: "Steep uphill for half an mile, but then things level out. I can do this!"

Resolve to spend quality time with maps and trail reports before venturing out on a new trail for this reason.

Be sure you know what the weather is going to be up to as well. (Chapter 6) A downpour can turn a tame trail into a quagmire. And you don't want to be hiking in an arroyo in a thunderstorm.

One last note: Seasonal variations will change your pace, too.

A crisp fall morning urges you to go faster than a muggy summer afternoon.

Tip: You will need more frequent breaks as the temperature swings away from moderate ranges: hot beverages and more snacks (Chapter 3) in cold weather, lots of water breaks and foot hydrotherapy (Chapter 4) in humid heat.

Hiking Pace In Groups

A quick word about pacing rules for hiking in groups.

The slowest hiker sets the pace for the group.

If you don't like that rule, don't hike with groups.

Harsh, but true. Why? Because it's good hiking practice to stay together, or at least stay in pairs, throughout a hike.

Having solo hikers strung out along the trail is asking for trouble, unless each of them is a strong, well-equipped hiker with navigating skills and buckets of common sense.

Too much can go wrong in the outdoors to allow an inexperienced, slower hiker to remain alone on the trail.

The trip leader should make the decision about whether the group splits up into smaller groups or not.

Putting the slowest hiker at the head of the line works well if the other hikers in the group are able to mentally adjust to a slower pace - without resentment or unkind comments.

And if *you're* the slow hiker, don't feel bad. Anyone who goes group hiking should be willing to accommodate the slowest hiker, and not get peevish about a slower pace. You are not "ruining" a hike with your slower pace.

So to sum it up: **Pacing on the trail is personal.** And it varies day to day, season to season, within your own body.

Be smart enough to avoid injury by being smart enough to allow your brain to acknowledge feedback from your joints, muscles, and bones. After all, they're doing all of the work!

Speaking of your body...

Shivers, perspiration and breathing rate: what they are telling you

Shivers are normal as you start down the trail on a brisk morning. Your skeletal muscles are trying to generate some extra heat for you.

Tip: It's okay to feel slightly cold for the first 10minutes of the hike, because you'll warm up quickly. And who wants to stop within 10 minutes and peel off a jacket? It completely destroys your pace.

However, if ten minutes come and go and the shivers continue, or are chased by intense sweating, it's possible you have a fever/chills cycle building up. You need to get off the trail ASAP and assess what's going on.

As you continue to hike after the warm up period, you'll feel sweat on your neck and back. Your breathing will get more labored.

Both of these are good signs. Your body is dumping excess heat generated by exercising muscles, and more breaths per minute brings more oxygen to your lungs.

Tip: There is an additional benefit of your muscular contractions during a hike: it gets the lymphatic system moving. That's another way to allow toxins and waste products to flow out of your open skin pores, where they can be flushed away when you shower or swim.

A few notes on coping with increased respiration rate:

*If you find yourself going into an open mouth breathing pattern, apply lip balm frequently to prevent drying out your lips.

*Lip balm with SPF of at least 5 will also prevent excessive UV radiation exposure to thin lip skin. Excess UV is a known trigger for "cold sores" (Herpes simplex viral outbreaks).

*Keep your mouth hydrated with frequent sips of water, or with hard candy to suck on. Chapter 3 Resources has some recommendations.

*Train yourself to breathe from your belly area, rather than using shallow upper chest breathing. This is more efficient in the long run.

STRIDE AND POLE ADJUSTMENTS

It's common to start off fast and hard, trying to maintain a certain pace throughout a hike.

Don't make that rookie mistake!

Stride adjustments are crucial responses to changing terrain and accumulating mileage.

Let's run (no, actually let's walk through) a few scenarios looking at how to use your stride and your poles to tackle the terrain.

Hiking Uphill

Consult the map before tackling steep inclines. How long will it last? How much gain per hour is expected?

This sets your internal timer with realistic expectations about what an ideal pace should be.

Before you begin an uphill section of the trail, sip a little water (Chapter 4), have a small carbohydrate-rich snack (Chapter 3), and stretch your thigh and butt muscles (Chapter 9).

Adjust your hiking poles so the hill-side pole is a bit shorter. This allows you to keep your stride equally balanced.

Tip: If your poles aren't adjustable, take your hand off the top of the hill-side pole and grip it lower down to make up the height difference. Some poles have fabric in just the right area for this purpose.

Use a "rest step" to gain elevation: Slow down so you can take shorter steps. Linger a bit over each step.

Your brain will be telling you that you'll never get anywhere at such a slow pace, but your muscles will thank you for giving them enough oxygen, and a brief pause from the contraction cycle, with each rest step.

If you feel that you need to take a break, it's best not to sit down. Your muscles will tighten up, and your mental perception of how far you still have to go uphill will work against you. Stand in one spot, bend over if you find it helps you catch your breath, and leave your pack on.

There's another factor that should be mentioned with tackling a steep elevation gain on a hike: the elevation you normally live and sleep at.

If you are a sea level woman trying to gain three thousand feet of elevation in one afternoon, your body will notice the decreased oxygen levels and make you breathe harder. This is normal, but annoying or distressing if you're not mentally prepared for it.

Give yourself plenty of time for the hike. Getting back to the trailhead via headlamp or flashlight is one way to buy yourself more time if your pace is slower than expected.

Or simply turn around, and try it again after you've spent more time at higher elevations.

Hiking Downhill

Tighten the laces on your footwear but give your feet enough room to expand from exertion. Avoid tight lacing up near your ankles because it impedes the return of blood to your heart.

If you have two pairs of socks on, and your toes are bumping the front of your boots, take off the less slippery pair to give yourself more room.

Check that your collapsible hiking poles are tightened up to bear weight on the downhill stretches.

Before you tackle the hill, stretch your thighs and calves, paying particular attention to your hamstrings (back of thigh) and gastrocnemius muscles (back of calves).

Spare your knees with a slow, steady downhill pace. The steeper the hill, the shorter the steps you should take.

Avoid the urge to lengthen your stride in response to gravity, because you can lose your footing and take a tumble.

Use your poles to minimize impact on your knee cartilage by planting one pole with each step. Allow your upper body to bear some of the strain.

Using poles can also give you confidence on a stretch of narrow rocky trail by adding stability to your stride. Just be sure the poles are sturdy enough (aluminum is less likely to snap than carbon fiber), and tightened up to prevent collapse.

Consider a knee brace if your knee feels unsteady or unstable.

Poles with shock absorption are worth the extra money because they absorb the jarring forces of each step before they vibrate up to your hands.

Sore tired hands at the end of a hike mean that you should be using shock absorbing poles. (It's also possible that your hand grips are too big for your hands.)

Breathing rate

Before you leave for the trailhead, check for tight clothing like a sports bra that restricts full breaths, or digs into your chest and back.

Adjust your backpack straps, especially the sternum strap across the top of your chest, to allow for more expansion of your rib cage without giving up a good fit.

You should be able to carry on a conversation with your hiking partner, or recite a poem to yourself, regardless of whether you're going uphill or downhill.

If you are laboring to catch your breath, your cardiovascular (heart and blood vessels) system is having a hard time working with your respiratory (lungs) system. This means that in the long run, you need more conditioning for the type of hiking you're doing.

This could also be a case of "early season breathing", and things will smooth out as the hiking season unfolds.

Short term, if you feel your heart pounding or you get hit with a wave of dizziness, you're not getting enough oxygen.

- Slow down.

-Sit down.

-Catch your breath.

-Don't give in to panic. This is fixable!

If you feel like you're going to pass out, sit down and put your head between your legs. Take slow breaths until the dizzy feeling passes. If you're heading to a higher altitude, turn around immediately.

Have you eaten and are you hydrated enough? Stop and fix the problem before continuing.

An aside about poles

Poles for hiking can be called hiking poles, trekking poles, hiking staffs, hiking sticks, and probably some other words I haven't run into yet.

You will run into hikers (just don't run over them) who scoff at the silly idea of using poles. Usually, those hikers have fairly young cartilage and are lean, energetic, and still believe in the invincibility of the human body.

But time has a way of erasing everyone's cartilage eventually. Why take a pounding on your precious joints even if you feel bullet proof right now?

Test it for yourself.

-Rent or borrow a pair of poles and hike a steep downhill section for at least half a mile.

-How do your knees and legs feel the next day?

An added benefit: using trekking poles provides a upper body workout. Why not tone your arms while you build lower body strength on every hike?

Another area of debate: use one pole, or two?

I've used just one pole, and my rhythm and balance feels "off". I've also noticed that the side of my body using the pole (usually my dominant right side) seems more tired after the hike.

Having only one pole also makes me feel as though I "over-reach" on downhill slopes, a balance problem best avoided.

Thus, I recommend using two poles. But again, experiment and see what *feels best for you*.

THE SOAKED SHIRT RULE

You won't find this rule in any other book, or anywhere on the internet, because it's one that Hiking For Her invented.

Soaked shirt rule for women: If you reach your dayhike objective and your shirt is completely soaked, back to front, top to bottom, you need to sit down and drink at least a quart of water before you do anything else.

Don't break or bend this rule, just do it.

As you sip, ask yourself these questions:

-Was I pushing myself too hard? Maybe a new hiking pace policy needs to be put in place!

-Is this shirt cotton? A bad choice for wicking perspiration and odor control! Resolve to buy a moisture wicking shirt for the next hike. (Chapter 1)

-Is the temperature/humidity too high for me today? Apply a moist cool towel on the back of your neck to start the cool down process.

Tip: During hot weather, start off with a frozen water bottle and use it as an ice pack to cool yourself down *at rest stops. Or you can buy a towel for this purpose – See Chapter 8 Resources.*

-Do I feel shaky? You need to eat carbohydrates (Chapter 3) after ingesting water. Your blood sugar level is probably a bit low.

-Should I have been drinking more water along the way? The answer is probably yes. You've sweated out lots of water, and haven't replenished it. But you're doing it now, right?

A few shirt tips:

*Always carry a dry shirt in your pack. Switch it out half way through your hike so you don't feel soggy and gross.

*A fresh shirt prevents chafing in tender damp places like armpits, beneath your breasts, and lower back.

*A dry shirt to change into is super important in cool windy weather, because your body temperature can tumble quickly and then you have to spend lots of calories warming back up.

*Have another dry shirt back at the trail head so you can go into town for dinner without any odor or stain worries. It also makes the ride home more pleasant.

Chapter 8 Summed Up

Who knew there was so much to learn about pacing yourself on a hike? Now you do!

This chapter covered the "Hike Your Own Hike" approach to figuring out an ideal hiking pace, and then how to adjust it as needed.

Did you notice that this chapter goes hand in hand with Chapter 4 on hydration? The Soaked Shirt Rule proves it.

You already know that perspiration is a great way to cool your inner core, and it's great for removing toxins from your lymph system and skin.

But now you can apply the soaked shirt when you seem to be sweating buckets.

Chapter 8 Take-Aways

Hike your own hike, even when it means disappointing or frustrating your trail buddies.

Find your personal hiking pace, knowing that it will vary with conditions and your body's cycles.

Downhill hiking is just as hard as uphill hiking, so **use your stride and trekking poles** for maximal comfort and support.

A soaked shirt indicates an **immediate need for hydration**. Sit, sip, and switch your shirt.

Chapter 8 Resources

Hiking For Her Recommendations for Pacing Help

POLES

I've tried several pairs of poles, but these are the ones that come along on every hike because they've proven themselves to be tough, easy to collapse or extend, and lightweight: Black Diamond Trail Pro Shock Trekking Poles, adjustable within a range of 68 – 140 cm.

SHIRTS

You have a lot of options, but it's best to stick with moisture wicking, fast drying fabrics.

Long sleeved shirts for cold weather should be able to wick away perspiration without leaving you a soggy mess. No tight cuffs or collars, please - I want my hiking clothing to provide me with full range of motion as I'm scrambling up rocks or snow banks.

That's why I prefer the easy pull-on style in hiking clothing. These also avoid the worries of a loose or missing button, or a broken zipper that catches on other clothing.

Short sleeved shirts are great for spring and fall layering under a jacket. Again, pull on styles are the way to go, with a V neck giving you the most room for movement.

I use sleeveless shirts in warm weather because I heat up quickly. I avoid tank top styles, because the narrow straps leave me vulnerable to chafing from my pack straps.

Tip: Always choose quick drying fabrics which accept spot removers without fading the fabric.

I find cotton to be too heavy, and not good at releasing moisture or odors. Also, cotton doesn't stand up well to the frequency of wash cycles each year I put my clothing through; it tends to fade and get misshapen.

It also hangs on to food spills and stains, outing me as a trail slob.

LIGHTENING UP THE GEAR

Ready to go light? Read the HFH article Ultralight Backpacking Gear: Weigh To Go!

Hiking For Her Additional Information

HIKE YOUR OWN HIKE

Read a free chapter in Francis Tapon's Hike Your Own Hike (Appalachian Trail saga) at http://francistapon.com

HIKING POLES AND SHIRTS

Read these HFH articles on the website:

Hiking Poles: Why Use Them

Shoulder Injury Prevention For Hikers

Womens Best Hiking Shirts

The Best Plus Size Womens Outdoor Clothing

UPF Sun Protective Clothing

After Your Hike

You've planned a great hike, using the first part of this book: Chapters 1 -5.

You've been out on the trail, having a safe and enjoyable hike thanks to Chapters 6-8.

Now you have to face the aches, pains, and unavoidable learning experiences that are part of the joy of hiking.

Don't worry, this section gives you a plan!

Chapter 9: Self Care

Chapter 10: Life Long Learning

Ready to wrap things up? Here we go...

Chapter 9: Hiker Self-care

Congratulations!

Now that you've read all the previous chapters, you are well equipped to plan and tackle the perfect day hike for your abilities and interests.

But a smart dayhiker also makes plans for the *post-hike hours,* as well as the recovery phase lasting into the next day and beyond.

You are definitely in the category of "smart" because you're reading this book. Just keep reading for some easy strategies to minimize your muscle soreness and recovery time.

These include:

-Anti-inflammatory actions

-Dealing with muscle soreness

-Stretching and conditioning

-Foot care ideas

-Attitude and motivation

HIKING SELF CARE: THE BIG PICTURE

Hiking self care is not something you see discussed very much in hiking magazines or blogs. I've often wondered about this.

Is it because hikers are tough and just "suck it up" when something hurts? Example: The expectation is that new boots will be painful, and you just have to suffer for awhile. Chapter 1 blasts that myth!

Or is it because nobody in the health care realm teaches hikers how to prevent problems before they start? You know how to prevent blisters, thanks to Chapter 6.

Could it be because it's just too time consuming to attend to sore muscles, hot spots on your feet, or signs that your pack is too (fill in the blank: big, heavy, small, tight)? After all, there's a hiking objective ahead, and you're burning daylight!

Hey! You already know how to deal with this, thanks to Chapters 1 and 6, so you are way ahead of the curve.

It probably doesn't matter what's behind why hiking self care is so often overlooked, but it matters a lot to me that *you* stay out of pain and remain happy on the trail.

That's why I'm sharing with you these easy, do-able suggestions for taking care of your hard working body once you leave the trail.

If some of these suggestions feel like tough love, they are!

Tip: You're worth it.

ANTI-INFLAMMATORY ACTIONS

FACT: Hikers use all of their muscles.

FACT: Working muscles can become inflamed.

That's exactly why *hiking inflammation* is a topic you need to be familiar with.

"Inflammation" used to describe a hiker's body implies that at least 2 of 5 known **"cardinal signs"** of inflammation are present: heat and redness, if not soreness, swelling or loss of function.

See how the name fits? Flames are hot, red and can be painful.

Cardinal signs after a hike give you a strong clue that you've overdone it.

So is inflammation a bad thing? Or is it helpful?

The answer depends upon your point of view.

-If you realize that inflammation is a non-specific, protective mechanism built into your body to deal with trouble before things get worse, you'll be thankful for it and work with it.

-But if you ignore it, argue with it, or suppress it, it's going to keep trying to get your attention until you finally acknowledge that there's a problem. Chronic inflammation will rob you of trail time.

Let's work with it, okay?

Anti-inflammatory suggestions

Previous chapters gave you some hints and tips for fighting inflammation. Now let's get really specific, with these easy to do suggestions.

Suggestion #1: Why wait for "the morning after" effect? Once you're back at the trail head, and your pack and boots are off, **do some pre-emptive stretches to loosen your muscles**.

Nothing fancy, just a little relief for the tight spots. Try this:

-For balance, grab the top of your hatch back, or the roof of your car, or a tree trunk, with your left hand.

-Put your other hand around your right ankle as you bend your right knee, bringing your foot as close to your buttocks as possible. Hold that position for the count of 10. Breathe deeply.

-Ahhh! Your muscles on the front of your right thigh say thank-you-very-much. And of course, you'll do the other side, too.

Don't forget the muscles on the back of the thigh!

-Find a slightly elevated rock or patch of ground. Put your left heel on it, point your toes toward your knee and lean in a bit until you feel a stretch in your thigh muscles.

-Hold for the count of 10, and then switch sides.

You probably think "This is too simple". Since when is simple bad?

Please believe me when I say that **simple beats complex** every time for prevention of hiking inflammation. All it takes is a little discipline.

And sometimes a memory jogger, like a sticky note on the dashboard: "Stretch before getting in!"

Stretching brings you peace of mind, and some cellular peace, too: it lengthens the muscles fibers, re-sets the muscle spindles, and generally tells the muscle cells that the hard work is over.

Suggestion #2: Ice down the area

Throw a cooler of ice and water bottles in the back of the car before you leave home, and enjoy the cold water as a refreshing part of the cool down routine after a long summer hike.

Use the ice filled cooler as a foot bath to head off hiking inflammation!

If that sounds too unsanitary, or takes too much planning, AND there's a convenient snow patch or rushing stream handy, plunge your feet and legs into there instead.

Or soak your bandanna until it's icy cold, and apply it to your usual trouble spots.

The point of hydrotherapy is to let Mother Nature help you out by reducing swelling and reversing congestion.

Ah! Icy cold water hurts so good! And it keeps hiking inflammation to a minimum.

If you have to wait until you're home, have some icing supplies ready to go.

-Freeze water in small paper cups before you leave for your hike. Peel off the top of the cup, and apply the ice to sore spots. Don't put the ice directly on your skin.

-For bumpy sore areas like your knees and elbows, wrap a frozen bag of peas in a thin towel and apply your home made compress to the sore area. Then eat the peas for dinner! Yum, complex carbs.

Suggestion #3: Ingest some **water and a carbohydrate rich snack** as soon as you get back to the trail head.

Along with replenishing your depleted nutrient stores, you can swallow an over-the-counter (non prescription) anti-inflammatory.

NOTE: This is not medical advice. Short term over the counter pain relief is a personal choice based on pre-existing medical conditions or any prescription medications you take. Consult your health care provider for advice.

Which anti-inflammatory to use? The general rule is that NSAIDS (aspirin, ibuprofen, naproxen) will relieve pain and swelling, while acetaminophen will suppress pain signals but not address inflammatory swelling.

Anti inflammatory topical applications are also useful. My favorites are Tiger Balm and Mineral Ice: fire and ice! See Chapter 9 Resources for full details.

Suggestion #4: A nice long **soak in a hot bathtub** saturated with Epsom salts (magnesium sulfate).

This is the cheapest way to buy relief from muscle pain and stiffness that I know of, and one of the best.

Non-soakers can use this technique by soaking a soft cloth in warm water saturated with Epsom salts, and applying it to the sore area.

See Chapter 9 Resources for more details on this low tech, inexpensive way to take care of sore muscles.

Suggestion #5: Hiking inflammation can be combated by ingesting anti inflammatory **herbs and spices**.

Throw yourself on the mercy of a trained herbalist here. Ask her for a list of herbs known to combat hiking inflammation.

Also ask for recommendations for herbal formulas designed to tackle inflammation. Be sure these won't interfere with current medications.

And in case you're not into natural remedies, where do you think aspirin, a famous anti-inflammatory, comes from? Willow tree bark! It doesn't get any more natural than that!

Food can also provide anti-inflammatory relief. Curcurmin in curry, cinnamon in your favorite cookie recipe, cherry juice ...explore the wonderful world of eating your way out of hiking soreness.

The Resource section at the end of this chapter will provide additional information on this approach.

Suggestion #6: Apply PRICE to your inflamed tissues. This acronym is a way to remember the basics of this approach.

Protection from additional injury.

Rest (I sympathize! You'd rather be hiking…).

Ice (apply an ice pack).

Compression (ace bandage, loosely applied to swollen area).

Elevation (not the trail kind, the lay on the couch and prop it up kind).

Sudden problems on the trail such as a popping sound, inability to bear weight, lots of pain and swelling, or numbness, require aggressive short term PRICE, followed by medical attention.

PRICE can also be used at home after a hike leaves you with signs and symptoms of inflammation. It's a low cost, thoughtful approach to helping yourself out of a painful situation.

Hiking inflammation suggestions, part two

To recap: Hiking inflammation is no joke.

It can come out of nowhere on a dayhike.

Or it can build up over time and create nagging chronic injuries in soft tissue. Those take a long time and lots of patience to heal.

If you're a young twenty-something of a hiker, you can probably get away with pushing through the pain and stiffness - for awhile.

But if your twenties are in your rear view mirror, it's time to pay attention to stiff, sore muscles and joints before their whispers turn into roars.

Make these **good hiking habits** part of your trail routine:

*Before your hike, drink water and eat a complex carbohydrate-rich breakfast.

*If you're a caffeine addict, realize that for every cup of coffee or black tea you consume, you lose more than that in water via urination. (Chapter 4, Hydration)

*During the hike, drink water and snack frequently to give your muscles the fuel they need.

*Take off your footwear, including socks, at least once during a long hike to allow blood circulation to normalize.

*Take advantage of hydrotherapy opportunities provided by Mother Nature: snow fields, rushing streams, cool mud, shallow lake shores.

*Pay attention to hot spots on your feet and deal with them immediately, because blisters suck. And the inflammation and open wounds they cause can set you up for a blood-borne infection (insert frowny face here).

*Stretch any cramped or complaining muscles as soon as you notice their complaints. Every hour or so, stretch your arms over your head and bend over to loosen your lower back. And don't forget to stretch at rest breaks.

*Take more frequent rest breaks toward the end of the day, when your muscles and joints begin to speak up.

*As you hike, breathe from your belly, not your upper chest. At a rest break, rest one hand on your chest and the other on your belly. Guess which hand should be rising high with each in breath?

*Make an anti-inflammatory regime post-hike just another part of your regular hiking routine.

To wrap things up, repeat after me:

An ounce of hiking inflammation prevention is worth way more than a pound of cure!

SELF CARE FOR MUSCLE SORENESS

Hiking soreness and pain: the price you pay, right?

Hey! You don't have to be fatalistic about how much pain and stiffness you have to endure the day after a hike. There are ways to stack the deck in your favor, and against muscle soreness.

How? By paying attention to **every factor you can manipulate** to avoid that hiking soreness. In previous chapters, you did just that, by looking at:

-properly fitted gear;

-correct weight distribution in your pack and through your spinal column, hips, and knees;

-adequately conditioned and warmed up muscles;

-adequate hydration and hiking food;

-correct hiking techniques for terrain and distance;

-ergonomic hiking aids like boot inserts and poles.

And you just read about lots of anti-inflammatory actions you can take.

Now let's get started on a closer look at the touchy subject of muscle soreness.

Warm up those muscles - and *then* GO

I know that it's a pain (pun probably intended) to add one more thing to your trailhead routine. Who wants to burn daylight standing around stretching?

And the danger of being mistaken for a yoga instructor is very real.

Tip: If you are one, hand out your business cards to passing hikers, advertising a "hiker special".

Stretching at the trailhead just makes sense. Here's why.

Muscles need a clue that you are going to use them to get to the top of that pile of rocks. Really, it's just a matter of simple courtesy because stretching delivers more blood to them, lengthens their fibers, and tells them to loosen up a little.

Alas, stretching weak muscles probably doesn't do much good, in terms of preventing muscle soreness.

While it doesn't have to take a lot of time and effort to begin to build more muscle strength, it does require new habits in your daily routine.

-Take the stairs and shun the elevator.

-Enjoy a brisk 15 minute walk at lunch time.

-Plan some sort of aerobic exercise (dance, brisk walk, run, bike, swim) of at least 30 minutes duration several times per week.

-Take a walk after dinner in place of your favorite TV show. Or maybe before it?

Just a note: Not everyone recommends stretching before a hike. If you're a limber twenty something who is into yoga, you can probably get away with skipping it.

Older and less flexible hikers would do well to pay attention to warming up before tackling the trail. It's a simple way to avoid injury and muscle pain.

Improve your muscle strength

It's a biological fact that strong muscles recover more quickly from exercise, burn fuel more efficiently during and after a hike, and make you feel more balanced (i.e. confident) on tricky footing.

The key to having muscles that don't ache like crazy after a hike?

Start somewhere, and (ok, you knew this was coming)... Just Do It!

You don't need a high powered fitness guru to help you. Put together your own personal strength program. You can start small, as outlined above.

But if you're committed to getting stronger, incorporate these habits into your life:

-Moderate, daily weight training

-Resistance exercises

-Daily walks of at least 60 minutes

-Swimming (especially in warm salt water if you have chronic pain)

-Biking or spin classes

-Yoga

-Dance or kickboxing classes.

Just as with your hiking pace, don't let anyone intimidate or push you into doing more than you feel you can handle at any one time. Set your own expectations, and be flexible about measuring your progress.

You'll know you're making progress with getting stronger when you push yourself a bit on the trail and you feel fine the next day.

That's something to celebrate, so hoist your water bottle in a toast to yourself. I'll be there with you in spirit.

Self-massage for sore muscles

Here's where I might lose you because I'm still not advising you to reach for the pain relief pills or a bag of ice.

Instead, I'm going to recommend self massage for your major muscle groups - at least the ones you can reach with your own two hands.

Depending on your familiarity with massage, I'm expecting one of two reactions: a groan ("*Isn't that vaguely inappropriate?*") or an enthusiastic nod of agreement followed by "*But I don't have time for that*".

Here's the beauty of **self massage for hiking soreness:** you have everything you need without opening your pack. Two hands, sore muscles, a commitment to self care ... what are you waiting for?

Start with your feet, even if they aren't sore.

-Examine the skin and nails, looking for blistered hot spots, long or torn nails, broken skin, calluses, fungal infections --- rule those out as sources of hiking soreness.

-Now, sitting comfortably, cup one foot between your two clean hands and probe gently for sore spots.

Self massage is the most effective for foot soreness, because you can give yourself immediate feed back on where and how much it hurts.

Let your intuition guide how much pressure to use and how long to work on each sore spot.

-If you have access to warm water, soak your feet before and after the massage (extra points for soothing aromatherapy scents such as lavender or rosemary added to the water.)

-While you're at it, sip some cool water to hydrate those loosening muscle fibers.

-Some hikers find it soothing to alternate warm with cool water foot soaks, ending with cool water.

-And if you have a favorite foot lotion, apply it while your skin is clean, soft and supple.

If you've never given your feet this much attention, please try it! You count on your feet to carry you on your hiking journeys, so pay them back with some love.

Now for the leg and thigh muscle groups that power you up the trail. Use the same basic approach to deal with hiking soreness that worked so well with your feet:

-Cup a calf or thigh muscle with both hands.

-Probe gently for the sore spots.

-Press down on them for as long as feels right. Don't be afraid to use lots of pressure. You are compressing the tissues, including the lymph channels, and helping clear out any congestion while redirecting it back to the heart.

-If you find exquisitely painful spots, use one thumb or knuckle to put direct pressure there. Let your pressure "sink in" as you breathe deeply, and don't be surprised as the pain diminishes. Be persistent but gentle. Give your muscles the time they need to "let go".

There's not much you alone can do about hiking soreness in your upper back, but you can certainly cup your shoulder in one hand and work out the sore spots, or rub your neck and lower back using slow circling motions.

Another trick: Lean back or lie down on a bumpy surface and use your body weight to press against the sore spots.

-Use old tennis balls or dog toys at home.

-Use a handy (did you miss that pun?) rock or log on the trail.

It's amazing how much better sore muscles feel after such gentle but sustained treatment. And directing your breath into the sore areas seems to help, too.

If hiking soreness is a **routine problem** for you, go to a professional licensed massage therapist and request the Hiker's Special: extra attention focused on the large working muscle groups that get you up and down the trail!

STRETCHES

Chapter 8 introduced the idea of stretching at the trailhead. It's included again here as an enticement to take it seriously.

As with all new habits, you've got to start somewhere.

I invite you to try this:

-Write yourself a sticky note and put it on your hiking gear. Guess which word you're writing on it?

-Once you get out of the car, you'll see the note and hopefully decide to start this new habit. Or at least give it a try.

Here's an easy introduction to best practices at the trailhead:

-Grab hold of the car (I use the hatch or trunk lid when it's open) with one hand.

-Bend your opposite knee and grab that ankle to pull it back toward your thigh (gently).

-Hold it for the count of 20.

-Feel that elongating muscle? If not, a bit more "oomph" in the pulling will do the trick.

-Now do the other leg.

-Shake both legs a bit to help drain the blood back to your heart.

Note: Never force a stretch. If your lower back is tight, or your thigh muscles just don't want to stretch, take a look at your daily non-trail habits.

-Do you sit for long stretches (Ha! Those darn puns) of time without a break?

-Maybe you need to set a timer to ring every 50 minutes so you can stand up to give your leg and back muscles some oxygenated blood.

Here's another easy stretch: Reach for the sky with both hands, then reach for the ground, clasp your hands together, and pull your arms downward to loosen your upper body.

Do this behind your body, too.

Other fast warm ups for muscles:

-Slowly bend over and touch your toes, or at least attempt to. This will "even out" the opposing muscles you warmed up above.

-Wiggle your toes before you cram them into your boots. They have muscles, too! Tiny little toe muscles need some love.

-Walk around on your tip toes, then on your heels.

-Doing a few ankle rolls, both directions, feels good, too.

Don't neglect your muscles once your pack is off at your lunch stop.

-Roll those shoulders.

-Try to touch your shoulder blades (scapulae) with your fingertips.

-Repeat the leg stretches outlined above.

Afraid you'll look silly? ***Who cares?***

You won't look silly when you blow past the non-stretchers as they slowly (perhaps painfully) lumber their way uphill!

If you think these stretches are too simple, too easy, or too much of a bother, ask yourself why simple and easy is a problem.

As for the "too much bother", what's up with that? As previously mentioned, you're worth the bother.

Because these quick "insurance policies" before and after a hike really do make a difference in diminishing next day soreness and in enhancing hiking performance.

You must trust me on this, young one.

FOOT CARE IDEAS

By now you've surmised that you shouldn't let your feet defeat you on the trail. And they won't, if you use these foot care ideas.

Proactive foot care strategies at home:

-Pick up marbles and straws with your toes while you read a book or consume electronic media.

-Walk barefoot on sand, grass and pebbles every chance you get.

-Try a foot reflexology path. (It will hurt the first time!)

-Apply firm, sustained pressure to sore spots on toes, arches and heels.

-Trim toenails before every hike.

-Before bed, do ankle rolls in both directions to send oxygenated blood to your feet.

-Ditch contortionist footwear forever: high heels, pointy toes, tight non-breathable shoes have got to go.

-Don't settle for "good enough" hiking footwear. Go for *amazing*.

Be proactive on the trail:

-Wiggle your toes vigorously every few minutes. Boots too snug for wiggling? You need a half size bigger.

-Sliding, bunching, pinching socks? Try a different boot/sock combo.

-Remove your boots and socks at rest breaks. Pull on your toes. Elevate your feet to aid the return of blood and lymph to your heart.

-To short circuit inflammation, plunge hot, swollen, achy feet into an icy stream, or use your bandanna or hat to create an impromptu cold pack from a snow field.

Swing into reactive mode for trail twinges, cramps and pain:

-Don't trudge onward without evaluating foot problems. It might be an easy fix: re-lace your boots, adjust your socks, or remove the pine cone from your boot.

-Muscle cramps indicate electrolyte depletion. Your nutrition and hydration strategies might need some tweaking.

-Don't ignore hot spots or that "uh oh" feeling in your feet. Traditional hiker fixes for hot spots (not actual blisters) include duct tape, band aids and moleskin.

-Blisters mean you've separated the top layers of skin from deeper layers, creating a nice little pocket for fluid to build up. Deal with a blister immediately with moleskin.

-The perennial blister question: To pop or not to pop? If you've got the supplies to do a clean job of it, popping might buy you some more trail time. Or it might buy you an infection with a deeply blistered area. Tough call.

-Achy feet could be due to "fallen" or "high" arches. Supportive and sturdy hiking boots with custom fitted arch supports (orthotics) might make your feet happier on the trail.

-Bruised, sore feet and toes indicate tight fitting footwear pressing on the underlying bones and soft tissues. Try bigger boots with thicker, more cushiony socks, combined with neatly trimmed toenails.

-"Plantar fasciitis" or "painful heel syndrome" are chronic problems with your heel bone (calcaneus) and its soft tissue called fascia. Don't keep hiking when this level of pain is sending you a warning message.

-Swelling, bruising, deeper skin color, heat or pain (either statically or during motion) indicate muscle/tendon inflammation in your foot. Get off your feet as soon as possible and apply PRICE.

ATTITUDE AND MOTIVATION

What you think influences how you feel on the trail. If you expect the trail to be hard and "take it out of you", that's what you'll experience.

For this reason, do everything you can to anticipate trail conditions. The previous chapters are brimming with suggestions on how to do that.

Pinpoint your weak areas, and go to work on strengthening your trail skills so you are as prepared as possible.

Realize that you will have to meet unpredictable challenges at some point in your hiking career. It's just part of playing the game of hiking.

If your response to challenge is anger, fear or anxiety, you will put yourself in a weakened position because your decisions will be colored by emotion.

However, if your attitude is "I can handle this", you will get yourself out of any jam. You might even enjoy the adversity!

Common sense underlies a good attitude, right?

All of the tips in this chapter rely upon you to pay attention and be willing to receive the messages your body is sending to your brain.

Yes, little postcards are exchanged between body and brain every single minute of your dayhike.

-Please don't deny that pain is a message to be heeded.

-That "gut feel" that something is wrong is your best friend when you're out on a trail - it's hard wired into your instinct for self preservation.

-And not wanting to take the time to re-lace a boot that's rubbing your ankle is saying something a bit unflattering about your trail priorities (or about your boundaries with impatient hiking buddies – see Chapter 8).

Attitude and motivation are best friends. Keeping a positive attitude when you feel like quitting a hike leads directly to motivating yourself to make the right decision based on facts.

Sometimes it makes sense to turn around when your feet hurt.

Other times pushing yourself past your comfort zone yields unexpected rewards and leads to greater self confidence.

Who's the authority on your attitude and motivation? You know the answer!

If you're in the habit of negative self talk (along the lines of "too slow", "so clumsy", "really out of shape", "getting too old for this"), get tough with yourself and eliminate the trash talk.

Replace the worthless trash talk with factual statements, such as "I can walk another ten minutes before taking a break", or "I will have to adjust my turn around time because my pace is less than anticipated today."

Don't make excuses. Instead, make notes of what you're going to work on to improve.

Never, ever compare yourself to any other hiker. It's your hike, your trail, your time and it's in your power to make the most of it.

What I'm trying to say is this: please make it a priority to **take care of yourself**, so you can relax and enjoy your outdoor adventures.

Just one last little dollop of tough love, from me to you. You deserve trail time, and don't you ever forget it.

Chapter 9 Summed Up

If you don't take care of your hiking self, who will?

That's right, it's up to you to claim responsibility for feeling good on, and off, the trail.

Previous chapters showed you how to take responsibility for your safety and comfort.

This chapter gave you ideas for addressing specific hiking issues which plague all athletes, like tight muscles, soreness, inflammation, and lack of motivation.

A strong hiker needs a strong body, but also pays attention to attitude and motivation. Now you have some tools to work with to get as strong as possible!

One of the best gifts you can give yourself right now is the time and space to hike your own hike.

Take care of your body and your attitude, and nurture your growing thirst for outdoor time.

Pay attention to the feedback your mind and body sends you.

Make the "*I'd rather be hiking*" slogan a way to judge the ways you invest your time each week. Hint: some of it should be in getting stronger and smarter as a hiker. Carve out time for yourself, and hit the trail.

Chapter 9 Take-Aways

Inflammation is a routine part of a hiker's life. Anticipate it, and deal with it right away.

Muscle soreness means you've given your body a great workout.

By working out regularly, you can **decrease your muscle soreness duration and severity**.

Stretch your muscles before you ask them to work hard on the trail.

Your trail happiness begins and ends – literally – at your feet. So send a lot of **regular TLC** their way.

Cultivate a **good attitude** about inevitable trail tribulations.

Motivate yourself to move beyond self-imposed limitations.

Believe in yourself.

Chapter 9 Resources

Hiking For Her Recommendations for Self Care

FIGHTING INFLAMMATION

There are easy, inexpensive ways to make your muscles feel better after a long hard hike.

Tiger Balm is sold in little glass jars with a tiger on the lid in case you didn't get the "tiger" part. It is applied to unbroken skin, and creates a sensation of soothing heat. The ingredients include topical analgesics (pain relief).

I use the "ultra strength" variety, but there are various formulations to try so see what works best for your level of inflammation.

Fair warning: there is a distinct odor to Tiger Balm, a menthol/camphor smell, but it's not unpleasant. And on the up side: it hasn't stained my clothing or towels.

Or you could use the opposite approach: get things cooled down with **Mineral Ice**.

This blue menthol gel is rubbed into unbroken skin and produces an instant numbing sensation (topical analgesic) to tackle the soreness in your muscles. I've used this when doing sports massage, with good results.

Be aware that it will diminish sensation in the application area, so don't try to do anything strenuous right after you apply it, or you could injure yourself.

With either of these products, **WASH YOUR HANDS** before touching your eyes or mouth, or you'll be sorry!

By relieving the muscle soreness, you are helping flush the muscles of lactic acid and other compounds produced during exercise. That's going to reduce the healing time between hikes, especially if coupled with proper hydration and good nutrients.

The cheapest source of anti-inflammatory muscle relief is applying old fashioned Epsom salts (magnesium sulfate) to the problem. Fill up a bathtub with warm water, mix in plenty of these salts, and soak until the water cools down.

STRETCHING

This is a habit that you have to build one hike at a time. And be sure to reward your good behavior with noticing how much less stiff and sore you feel!

Read the HFH articles Back Stretches, Hiking Back Pain, and Sore Feet After Hiking.

FOOT CARE

Massage lotion

Aveeno makes nice fragrance free skin products for foot massages.

They tend to be non-greasy and stay put when your skin sweats.

Hiking For Her Additional Information

FOOT CARE

The Institute for Preventive Foot Health offers common sense foot hygiene tips.

INJURY PREVENTION

This HFH article give you additional insight into hiking aches and pains, with lots of links to specific body areas (neck, arms, etc.): Injury Prevention

HIKING WITH CHRONIC PAIN

Read the HFH article Hiking And Arthritis.

Visit the Arthritis Foundation and enter the search term "hiking"

Chapter 10: Keep Learning

In Chapter 1 – 9, you learned the *basic physical requirements* for a dayhiker, including:

-comfortable **footwear,**

-a **backpack** to **carry Ten Essentials,**

-**food and hydration** that works with, not against, you on the trail,

-a **hiking clothing system** to layer on and off,

-and a **destination,**

-with a **plan to get there and back safely.**

We also explored the ***mental requirements to keep yourself going strong:***

-**motivation** and **a good attitude,**

-**common sense,**

-**first aid** and **navigation** knowledge,

-a dedication to **self care,** and

-**self awareness.**

But to be honest, a strong hiker never stops learning, whether by accident (literally) or by design.

Wouldn't you rather *design* your own learning opportunities?

I thought so, which is why Chapter 10 is right here for you.

Enjoy browsing through these life long learning resources for hikers. Then pick one, and give your brain something new to learn.

LIFELONG LEARNING: A HIKING BEST PRACTICE

Whew! You've done a lot of reading about how to be the best dayhiker you can be.

Nine chapters in all.

Now it's time to put down the book and hit the trail.

But just a heads up: Expect to be challenged with a few of Mother Nature's pop quizzes.

You never know what she's got cooked up for you on a hike: weather hazards, animal encounters, gear failures, a skinned knee, navigational challenges - just to name a few likely scenarios.

Mom is a tough teacher, but you'll grow to respect her lessons. Each one provide an opportunity to test your current knowledge, while pointing out your knowledge deficits.

Don't take it personally! Every hiker gets less than perfect scores at various points along the hiking trail of life.

So don't put down this book quite yet.

Soak up the resources Chapter 10 provides for you.

And keep this book handy as you gain trail experience. When you get some feedback pointing out a knowledge deficit, consult the right chapter in this book for hiking advice and suggestions for how to solve your specific trail problems.

Hikers who keep learning never fall out of love with hiking, and that's a fact.

HIKING RESOURCES FOR LIFE LONG LEARNING

Trail knowledge can come from many sources. As you hike, keep your eyes and ears open for Mother Nature's lessons.

For example, watching how a determined chipmunk gets into your pack can be a powerful lesson in why you should never give up.

So can forgetting your rain gear in an epic downpour.

Chapter 10 gives you suggestions for multiple sources of trail wisdom. Every learning channel is tapped in these resources and recommendations: visual, auditory, and kinesthetic.

Note that I only recommend what I feel is valuable and worth your time.

And just to mix things up a little, this chapter won't have a Resources section, because you're already in it!

Books For Hikers

The Hiking For Her website has book reviews you can dip into when you need a bit of inspiration, or a chance to see how other hikers approach the trail. Use these titles as key words to find the reviews:

*Married To The Trail (Continental Divide)

*When Grandma Gatewood Took A Hike (children's book with great illustrations)

*1001 Ways To Live Wild

Other books you might like:

*Becoming Odyssa: Epic Adventures on the Appalachian Trail

*Grandma Gatewood's Walk: The Inspiring Story of the Woman Who Saved the Appalachian Trail

You can find more recommendations on goodreads.com and booksforhikers.com

That should hold you for awhile, no?

Hiking Resources: Movies

Watching other hikers can inspire, amaze, tantalize, and scare you into hiking best practices.

Not to mention entertain you during the months when your favorite hiking trails are inaccessible.

And they can act as wonderful hiking resources for your upcoming trips, giving you a glimpse of what it's like to walk in another hiker's shoes.

If you're interested in Pacific Crest Trail (PCT) hiking, watch Tell It On The Mountain. There's a review of this movie on the HFH website.

If you're hankering after an Appalachian Trail (AT) experience, head over to the appalachiantrail.com website and search for their Top 10 movie list.

Just add popcorn.

Enjoy!

Gear Tips & Reviews

It's good hiking practice to read a few reviews before you purchase a big ticket item like a backpack.

But they're just plain fun to read any time you're considering a new piece of hiking gear.

The HFH website has gear reviews that are thorough, honest and fair. Just search for "gear review" and they should pop up.

I strive to give you balanced information so you can make an intelligent decision about the gear you need versus the gear you want.

Or use "best tips" to search the website for more ideas.

Other sources for hiking gear reviews:

-Gear Junkie

-Outdoor Gear Lab

-Gear Institute

Gifts For Hikers

You want to create a **"hiking gifts** wish list" to leave lying around (in)conspicuously.

Or perhaps you want to become known in your hiking circle for your great taste in hiking gifts.

Either way, visit the HFH site and search for "gifts". There's even a page for a non-hiker to come up with the perfect gifts for hikers.

Magazines For Hikers

Magazines are great places to get a monthly (daily??) trail fix when the weather is too nasty, or your schedule is too brutal, to get outside.

And hiking magazines can be great gifts (see above).

Autorenewal is the way to go if you don't want to pay the single copy newstand price.

And auto-renewal means no guess work about which issue(s) might be lost if you don't renew on time. I hate it when my subscriptions lapse and I have to pay full price for an issue.

Caution: Beware the lure of the glossy magazine ads!

But do use their annual Gear Guides or featured items as a road map of gear to consider.

Here are a few magazines pitched at us outdoorsy types.

Backpacker

Why I recommend it:

An obvious choice in the list of magazines for hikers, right?

I stopped subscribing to this magazine years ago, mostly because it didn't seem relevant to an aging hiker.

I gave it another look recently, and signed up for a subscription for 2 reasons: because I want to support print media which addresses the concerns of hikers, and because I can see myself getting value out of *some* of the content.

For instance, the Nature section is quite extensive.

You might enjoy the "Find hikes near you" feature using your zip code (on line version).

I also like the fact that they pay attention to changing environmental and climate issues.

They write about plants, animals, and wildlife destinations in addition to hiking trails and the latest gear.

Also, they seem to have a basic understanding that hikers come in two genders. But they do seem blind to the reality of older hikers. Baby steps, I suppose.

So Backpacker deserves a place on my "Magazines for Hikers" list.

However, a few cautions...

Cautions:

Their gear reviews are useful, but should be taken with a large grain of salt when the latest cutting edge (and pricey) stuff is featured on the page facing the review.

If the writing gets a bit too enthusiastic, beware! Remember that advertisers, not outdoor enthusiasts, keep this magazine afloat.

Because they try to appeal to a general audience, some of what they say won't apply to you. Grab the good stuff and let the rest roll right off your cortex.

Sometimes the writing gets a bit breathless and cutesy, which may become annoying.

To see if this hiking magazine is a good fit for you, go to the nearest public library and leaf through a current copy. I'm sure there will be one of those little postcards stuck in the magazine, offering THE deal of the century for a subscription!

Backpacking Light

Why I recommend it:

Lightening up on trail gear is something every hiker can strive for, and these folks dish the dirt on exactly how to make that happen.

They've been around for awhile, too, and have an established reputation as a "go to" source.

You can read forum posts and article summaries free of charge, and can join without paying to make your own comments.

For a minimal fee each month, you candownload print articles. It's like a "do it yourself" hiking magazine!

If you'd like to subscribe for deeper access to the archives, you can do so on an annual or lifetime basis (now there's a tricky calculation!).

Cautions:

This does not technically belong in the "magazines for hikers" category, because their offerings are set up more like a buffet/smorgasbord.

They're adamant about weight being the most important feature of a great hiking trip. If you're more relaxed about your pack weight, maybe this isn't for you.

High Country News

OK, I'm guilty. I called this one a magazine, when it's self-described as "a bi-weekly newspaper that reports on the West's natural resources, public lands, and changing communities".

Why I recommend it:

What I like about this publication is the wide range of writing styles and its coverage of topics important to any outdoor advocate (that includes hikers, right?).

I've learned a lot about the changing weather patterns that affect hiking, about the environmental disasters that impact trails, and lots more.

You can dabble for awhile with their free weekly newsletter before you commit.

Cautions:

It's aimed squarely at people residing in the western states of the USA, so if you're not hiking there, or don't plan to, it's not for you.

They cover politics, energy, industry and other topics that at first glance seem off topic for a hiker (although these things influence our ability to access trails, right?)

Don't expect trail reports, gear reviews or hiking snack recipes. But you will read about endangered wildlife, land use decisions and other things that a hiker might be interested in.

Snowshoe Magazine

If you're into snowshoeing, you might like an entire magazine devoted to your favorite type of winter hiking. You will find all sorts of wintery information, from beginner advice to adventurous snowshoe destinations such as Greenland.

Get Out There Magazine

Here's one that you have to sift through to get to the gold nuggets for hikers.

It's free, it's online, and it's geared toward young runners, bikers & winter sports enthusiasts.

However, there are gear reviews, tips for self care, and possibly some tantalizing new opportunities to use your hiking body in a new way hidden in the pages.

Adventure Journal

Here's the new kid on the block (June 2016), and will only be available in print. Retro, or what?

Because the magazine content won't be available on line, you might want to take a look at this publication with a single copy.

You can also sign up for their daily news feed, with links to great photos and intriguing articles.

Trail Groove

You have two options with this on line magazine:

a) free subscription, delivered monthly.

b) premium subscription which includes goodies like gear deals, give-aways, bonus material, and the satisfaction of supporting a hiking magazine.

Each edition features trail and trip reports, gear reviews and gorgeous photos. Their forum is a great place to get, and give, advice.

U.K. Magazines for Hikers

I won't pretend to know much about these magazines, but they do look intriguing.

Trail Magazine

The Great Outdoors Magazine

(I've got to admit that "hill walking" is a lot classier hobby to claim than "hiking".)

Australian Magazines For Hikers

Great Walks publication provides all the usual features for hikers: how to articles, gear reviews, news of upcoming events, suggestions for walks (a.ka. hikes), and photo contests.

You can sign up for their free newsletter, or look through their online articles.

And a subscription might be just the ticket for a fresh look at the sport we enjoy throughout the world!

Good General Hiking Resources

New to hiking? Information from the American Hiking Organization can get you started! They tend to avoid jargon and acronyms, making it easier to figure out how to apply their information to your style of hiking.

The Washington Trails Association (WTA) is aimed at one particular place in the United States, but has archived articles applicable to every hiker. Find this wealth of information at wta.org

I sincerely hope you find the entire Hiking For Her website a good general hiking resource.

To navigate through the hundreds of pages of tips and techniques, be sure to locate the Site Map button in the navigation bar.

Or go directly to the Resources page for lots of links to quality hiking information.

And don't forget that you can contact me with your specific questions. I read, and reply to, every email because I believe that as a life long learner who also happens to love to hike, it's important to share what I'm learning.

THE END – OR IS IT?

Congratulations! You've found the end of the best hiking tips for women dayhikers.

False alarm!

You can access all of the latest hiking tips from Hiking For Her in lots of different ways. Shall I count them for you?

*Use a free RSS feed to get the newest pages delivered to you like a virtual daily newspaper. You can sign up for that service on the HFH navigation bar on any page on the website.

*Contact me directly (diane@hiking-for-her.com) with your comments, suggestions and questions.

*If you'd like to stay current on hiking news, sign up for **Happy Trails**, a free monthly newsletter. Here's how one reader describes it:

> *"I just want to thank you for the dedication and care that you put into your website and newsletter.*
>
> *It's always a treat to see the latest newsletter in my inbox. Always informative and inspiring!" -Christina*

*Try **Trail Mix**, HFH's monthly collection of great hiking tips, give aways, and more.

*Cruise for some interesting pins on the Hiking For Her Pinterest page.

*Drop by the HFH Facebook page for a dose of inspiration.

*Enjoy a variety of seasonally appropriate hiking photos on the Hiking For Her Instagram page.

*Or see what else has been published on the HFH Amazon Author or Goodreads page.

*And make it a weekly habit to browse the Hiking For Her site, using the site map and search box to navigate.

In closing, I'd like to leave you with a quote:

*"**Nothing is more terrible than activity without insight.**"* -Thomas Carlyle

So when you find yourself having a less than enjoyable hike, pay attention to all of the factors we've covered in this book.

Ask yourself: What can you change? Adjust? Let go of?

And where can you learn how to do that?

Hint: You're holding the answer.

Don't forget, the flip side is just as true! When you have a spectacularly fun hike, what made it that way?

Take notes, jot down ideas, pay attention to yourself enjoying the trail. Your insights make the trail just that much more rewarding.

Because a thoughtful hiker is a successful, safe, happy and enthusiastic hiker.

May it be ever so for your happy trails.

SECRET BONUS CHAPTER!

Hikers are amazing creatures.

Female hikers, even more so.

So to help you get onto the trail in amazing comfort and confidence, here's a bonus chapter on how to buy a perfect day pack.

Enjoy!

How to Find the Right Pack

Grandma Emma Gatewood hiked the Appalachian Trail using a sack slung over her back, and it worked just fine for her!

But most hikers today would prefer to use a fitted backpack to carry the 10 Essentials (Chapter 2).

You are probably in agreement.

The problem is, not all packs are created equal. This makes it tough to figure out exactly *which* pack is going to be best for your trail use.

But all is not lost.

There's a strategic approach to gear shopping, and I'm going to share it with you right here: How to Find the Right Pack, in five easy steps.

To make the most of your time, I'll give you hints on day packs as well as backpacking packs. My prediction? You'll morph into a backpacker one of these days, if you aren't one already.

The trail calls, and we must answer.

By the time we're finished with this bonus chapter, you'll have answers to three important questions:

-Which *elements* of a pack should I look for?

-Which *features* are most important for me?

-Which pack should *I* buy?

Here's a quick preview of what you'll be learning: elements and features.

To be considered trail worthy, a backpack needs to boast these *elements*:

-durable,

-weatherproof,

-lightweight,

-affordable, including a decent warranty against constructive defects.

Plus, it needs built in *features* such as

-An ergonomic design to protect and ventilate your back

-Adequate capacity in convenient compartments to accommodate the 10 essentials plus your "must have" items

-Personalized features such as tailored torso length

-Dimensions which fit your body type and hiking style

In order to find the pack that will perform well and give you maximum comfort, you can use what I call the "5 easy steps".

That doesn't imply that finding a pack will be effortless.

In fact, these steps will ask you to do a bit of work, as in:

-introspection,

-research,

-planning,

-shopping, and

-making a final decision.

Let's get started!

Step One: A Bit of Introspection

It would be a mistake to think that one pack is going to meet all of your needs as a hiker.

It's also a mistake to listen to the hype and hysteria surrounding new product releases each year.

If you read hiking magazines (Chapter 10), you'll see lines like: "Best pack *ever*!!"

The question is, best pack for whom?

There's middle ground (and the perfect pack for you) out there somewhere, and we're going to find it.

To begin, please take a few moments to answers these questions:

How long have you been hiking?

Define "hiking" as any time spent this way: walking/tramping/wandering/exploring outdoors, as long as you were using your own legs for transportation.

-If your answer is "Never been hiking" or "Not long", you're in that delightful phase of falling in love with hiking.

I envy you!

You're in for a grand adventure.

-If you've been hiking for a few months to a few years, you already know the woes of improperly fitted or inadequate gear.

That's probably why you're reading this!

I won't let you down, I promise.

What is the average length of a hike for you?

-A hike or ramble of only a few hours probably means you don't need much in the way of heavy water bottles or vast amounts of food. Or maybe it does, if you're exploring territory that can turn against you quickly in cold weather.

-A typical day hike lasts 4-8 hours (or longer, if long daylight hours are available). You're going to need 10 essentials + food + water. These all add up to weigh you down.

-If you're an overnighter, you will have to add camping gear to your pack. Think of this as survival gear (shelter, heat source, water purification) but also think of comfort gear (a pair of base camp shoes to rest your sore feet, for instance).

-Multi-day trips require a pack that can stand up to abuse, weather, repeated access on dusty or wet trails, accidental dunkings in fresh or salt water, the random attack by famished squirrels, and more.

How many times per year will you use this pack?

-If you're just easing into the sport of hiking, be honest and admit that this particular pack won't see much trail dirt.

No worries! There's plenty of time to use it next year, and the next year.

-If you're a moderate hiker, a typical answer is in the range of 12 to 24 days per year, and mostly on week-ends with maybe one longer trip each year.

-Anything above 24 days/year puts you in the "heavy usage" category, from the perspective of a pack maker.

You need something bigger, more durable, weatherproof, and low weight. And don't forget comfort during high mileage days on the trail.

What's the most ambitious hike/hiking trip you're planning this year?

-You can always under-pack a pack, but can't do the opposite without sacrificing stability and performance.

So think about whether you should buy a pack that's just a bit larger than your current needs.

-The amount of gear needed translates into weight. Your pack must be able to handle the gear without compromising your stability, ergonomics, and comfort.

-If you want to do lots of elevation gain and loss, you'll have to pack your pack correctly so the load doesn't slide around or pull you off balance. You'll need the right pack for the job.

What is your age and body type?

-A long and lean hiker has a torso length quite different from a short curvy hiker. The range of 15 – 20 inches works for most females.

-A strong 20-something parent of toddlers might want to haul bigger loads than a 65+ year old.

-The dimensions of the pack need to provide adequate storage, hauling capacity, ventilation, and expandability for your body type. And not one drop extra, or you'll regret wearing it.

What is your budget? (not your "someday" budget, your actual one)

Which of these thoughts fit you best?

-No sticker shock, please!

This means you can't fathom why some packs are so darned expensive. The lowest price always gets your attention.

-I'll pay for essential elements and important features.

This means you've saved up for this pack and are ready to invest in it – after you examine it thoroughly.

-I need a pack right now, and I'm willing to pay for it.

You are more of an impulse buyer, or you've got a hike coming up fast.

Q & A is over now! Wasn't that fun?

Your replies to these questions have given you some insight into where you should enter the swiftly moving stream called "Buying a Pack".

You can tiptoe in and stay in the shallows until you get used to the water.

You can wade out into the middle and feel the current tug against you, but remain stalwart.

Or you can plunge in and see where you end up!

Which leads us to Step Two…

Step Two: A Bit of Research

Now that you're armed with your personal hiking profile, you can use the resources I provide to explore all of the pack options available to you.

There are many ways to learn about backpacks.

An Internet search for backpack manufacturers is a good place to start.

But a word of caution first.

Depending on which country you live in, outdoor gear company products may or may not be available. Or at least not readily available to *you*!

Maddening, isn't it?

Case in point: Amazon will not ship everywhere in the world.

So don't waste time on the Internet sizing up packs that you won't be able to buy, or will have to pay extra to obtain.

When you do a search for "backpacks", be sure you narrow your search criteria to include your specific location if there's any doubt in your mind about availability.

Another logical starting point is hiking magazines.

You might be tempted to jump onto hiking magazine websites, or pick up that glossy hiking magazine on the newsstand to read the backpack ads.

Nothing wrong with that, but please fire up your inner skeptic first. Ads are designed to do one thing, and one thing only: sell you a product.

If you're looking at ads, or "gear reviews" disguised as ads, you're not going to get unbiased information.

My advice is to avoid the pretty pictures and glowing adjectives, and cut straight to the chase: gear specifications ("specs") located on gear labels or manufacturer's websites. These are the objectives facts about that particular piece of gear: size, weight, materials, and other important details you need to make a good decision.

Brands that I trust due to years of trail use include:

-Deuter

-Osprey

-Kelty

-REI

-North Face

You won't go wrong starting your search for the perfect backpack with these names.

Once you've located some retailers offering you an array of packs, brace yourself for some jargon.

Every sport has its own vocabulary, and backpacks are advertised with words that might seem impenetrable at first glance. Here are a few examples to get you started:

-attachment point,

-ripstop Denier nylon, with various numbers attached (1200 is really heavy duty)

- access points: top, panel, hybrid

-style: alpine, traditional

-capacity (volume) in liters

-torso length

There's no room here to go into all of the details. Your best bet is to make a list of any words you don't understand, and read the manufacturer's specifications to figure them out.

Also make it your mission to read reviews.

The REI website, as one example, provides detailed customer feedback. You can learn a lot about a pack by reading those, so please take notes and read carefully.

On to the next step...

Step 3: A Bit of Planning

Before you begin to hunt seriously for a pack, dump all of your hiking gear in a pile in the comfort of your living room.

Add whatever water bottle(s) or hydration system you use, plus your lunch sack and other consumables (hygiene kit, for instance).

That's roughly the size of a pack you're looking for.

Some things you can squash down into a smaller footprint. Others you can't. But it's a good estimate.

There are seasonal variations to your gear pile, of course.

Example: Two water bottles for hot weather instead of one in winter.

Or a water filter to eliminate the extra bottle.

Now get out a metric tape measure and take some measurements: length, width, and depth of gear pile.

This gives you **volume**, which is a cubic dimension - as you just proved.

Note that many gear companies put the volume right in the pack's name. For example, the XXX SuperDuper Combo48 can be translated as "a volume of 48 liters", and can probably handle multi-day trips because of its size.

You guessed it! The bigger the number, the more you pay, so be sure you're in the correct range for your particular hiking plans. You want to avoid the "bigger is better" syndrome.

The right pack is just big enough (Baby Bear from the 3 Bears story would agree).

Don't set foot in a gear store, virtual or actual, without a volume number in mind. It is incredibly easy to be seduced by the rows upon rows of packs in every size, color and variety. (Trust me on this).

And if you are easily overwhelmed, it is important to go shopping with a few brands of packs already in mind (see above).

Otherwise, your plan devolves into asking whatever harried salesperson happens to be around. S/he will try to sell you a personal favorite, or show you a few possibilities, but when it comes time to make the choice, it's pretty much up to you.

And if you're on line shopping, you're really on your own.

So make a list, and use it as a guideline.

Let's rehearse your shopping approach: virtual –vs- bricks and mortar store.

VIRTUAL SHOPPING APPROACH

Brew a cup of tea or pour a refreshing glass of iced tea (depending on your location and season).

Have some snacks handy to keep your blood glucose levels on an even keel. Your neurons are going to be sucking down glucose like you wouldn't believe.

Be sure your work station (table, computer, chair, light source) are all adjusted for minimum eye strain. You might be sitting for a few hours and nothing is worse than getting tired before making a final decision. You want your time investment to pay off in the perfect pack.

Fire up your favorite Internet browser.

Enter the appropriate search terms: hiking gear, backpack, day pack, or the name of a particular brand you're interested in (which you identified in Step 2).

Narrow down your search to the pack's volume in liters.

For each website you visit, don't forget to poke around in the "clearance" section. The perfect pack might be last year's model, marked way down and waiting just for you.

Open up separate windows for each store/website so you can click back and forth between pack possibilities. This won't work with more than 2 or 3 packs at a time, unless you like feeling dizzy.

If there is a "compare packs" feature, use it! See Step 4 for some hints.

BRICKS & MORTAR STORE SHOPPING APPROACH

Prepare for your shopping trip as if you're going hiking.

That means load up on adequate nutrients, hydrate yourself, and pack (Ha! A hiking pun) a few snacks.

Why?

You do NOT want to run out of brainpower before you purchase your pack.

I don't know about you, but low blood sugar leads to reckless, "let's just get this over with" decisions that may be regretted later on the trail.

Wear or bring the hiking socks & footwear you'll be using with this pack. If this makes you squeamish, as in "I don't want to be seen in this store wearing my boots", that's an interesting factoid about your hiking self. File it for later examination.

Wear pants, skirt or shorts which give you good mobility and don't impede your ability to move your hips and knees.

If your hair is long, put it up. You don't want it to get caught under straps or in zippers.

Step 4 is all about how to maximize your shopping time investment.

Step 4: A Bit of Shopping

VIRTUAL SHOPPING

Once you land on a page featuring packs, use the search options to narrow your choices to exactly what you want: brand, size, price, and whatever other criteria are most important to you (color comes to mind).

Specify women's packs if possible.

Tip: You want ergonomic straps that fit female shoulders without mashing breasts or chafing armpits. Look for an S-shape designed to fit your curves.

You should be rewarded with just a few packs to consider.

If you're lucky, the website will allow you to do a side-by-side comparison of the packs you've chosen. It's very illuminating to do this, because you might identify features you didn't realize were important to you until you see them.

Or you might decide that the price point you want is too steep and you can give up a few features.

So don't skip a "compare" feature if it's available.

If you're unlucky, you'll have to create a spreadsheet for yourself in order to compare packs.

Populate the spreadsheet with the data you're gathering on each pack.

Be sure to fill in each pack's data completely, because you never know which items will be the tipping point for you and it's a pain to have to go back and look at each page again.

To get you started, here are some criteria for your spreadsheet:

-capacity, in liters,

-weight (ultralight, etc.)

-access point (top, panel, hybrid),

-top "lid" (fixed, floating, removable),

-suspension (fixed, adjustable),

-hip belt dimensions and padding (some are removable),

-back style (foam, mesh),

-frame style for backpacking packs only (internal, external),

-brand,

-price,

-warranty/return policy,

-possible adjustments (Velcro torso length, hip belt diameter, sternum strap),

-number of compartments

To be honest, I'd recommend some online reconnaissance prior to an "actual" shopping trip (see below).

As you can see, there are a lot of things to think about!

BRICKS & MORTAR SHOPPING:

You do have your list and/or spreadsheet in your hand, don't you?

And a pen?

Make a beeline for the pack department, and scope out any available salespeople.

You shouldn't need much advice from them at this point, but you might have questions about upcoming sales, current sales and coupons, or the ability to order a pack if it's out of stock.

It's good to make eye contact and exchange greetings so you have a social baseline to build upon.

If you have questions about return policies or exchanges, now it the time to ask. You don't want to wait around for a busy salesperson to have time for you once they're mentally finished with you.

Next, look for a full length mirror in the pack department, or close by.

You want to see how the pack rides on your back, and you want to be able to reach for, and tweak, the straps once you're wearing it. Unless you have eyes in the back of your head, you'll need a mirror to negotiate an unfamiliar pack.

Does the store have an indoor "track" of some sort, where you can walk around wearing the pack?

Do they provide bean bags or other labeled weights to put inside?

Did you remember to wear the socks and boots you hike in?

Finally you can begin to look at the packs!

If you're a brand shopper, locate your favorite.

Only do one brand at a time, or you'll get confused about which pack had which features.

Use the product tags to find the correct dimensions and capacity.

Before trying on a pack, take a close look at the workmanship (or lack thereof). Here are a few questions to help you judge quality.

-Is this pack constructed from water and abrasion resistant materials which can be waterproofed, such as Cordura, packcloth, or ripstop nylon?

-Is the stitching applied with strong thread (nylon for highest strength), around 6 -10 stitches per inch? Once you pass a certain price point, seams and stress points should be reinforced with extra stitching.

-Are there dangling threads on the seams? This might indicate sloppy craftsmanship.

-Are the zippers plastic "coil"? You want them to stand up to grit, tugging and weather extremes over many seasons.

-Finally, ask yourself: "Is this a color I can live with?" Some women like to stand out on the trail, others prefer to blend in. Let your gut tell you if the burnt orange is a deal breaker or not.

Now pick up the pack to get a feel for its heft and dimensions.

What do you notice about the straps?

Open up the straps to their fullest extent and put on the pack.

You should have immediate feedback in terms of the pack size.

-Does it overwhelm your frame, as happens frequently with petite hikers?

-Does it fail to cover your back and seem too short on your torso?

-Are your arms squeezed by the straps?

Pay attention to what your body tells you about this pack, before you make any adjustments.

Now put the pack on your back.

How does the pack sit on your hips?

-If it's too big, it misses your hips and aims for your thighs.

-If it's too small, it's on your waist rather than your hips.

Adjustment time!

If you're not familiar with how to adjust the pack, ask for help from the salesperson. Or start tugging on straps and use the scientific method to keep track of cause and effect.

Better yet, press the trail buddy you've brought along into service.

Have them adjust all of the straps you can't reach, and let the mirror guide you in deciding if the straps are too snug, too loose, or just won't work for your body dimensions.

Walk around in the pack, noting any points of tugging or slipping.

If something feels tight, re-adjust the straps and stride around, using the gait you'd use on the trail.

You will know when the pack tries to fight you, or when it works with you.

Sure wish I could be right there with you!

But if you've done the previous steps, you should have enough data to make an informed decision about the pack: either it goes back on the rack, or it goes home with you.

Don't forget to inquire about the return policy, just in case this isn't the pack of your dreams.

Step 5: A Bit of Decisiveness

Regardless of your shopping location, you should have whittled your decision down to one or two, at most three, packs.

Now it's "fine tooth comb" time, meaning that you've got to go back over the pack(s) again, but with ruthlessness used only in card games and spring closet cleaning.

Ask yourself:

-Are you a gentle hiker, never dumping your pack in mud or snow?

-Do you get tangled up in thick brush, sit on pine pitch, or scoot over abrasive surfaces?

-What are the odds that your pack will never be insulted with pelting rain or a mud splashes?

-Is your perfect trail root and rock free, with a low elevation gain? Or is it a humdinger straight up the rocks to some spectacular spot, requiring lots of sweat and uphill perseverance?

The pivotal question underlying all of the above questions, and which you must answer, is:

"Can this pack stand up to whatever hiking conditions I'm going to throw at it?"

Maybe you don't know exactly what's in store for you, right?

If you're just getting started on this whole hiking thing, you'll want to proceed cautiously. Stick to marked trails, hike with at least one partner, and don't load up with unnecessary gear.

A low end pack is just what you need right now.

However, you might want to think about the wisdom of buying a mid-range pack that will last long enough to hold up while you develop your hiking skills. You don't want to "outgrow" a pack too soon, in the sense that it's not durable enough, or its capacity is too small, after one hiking season.

The opposite mistake is also possible.

-Don't buy a pack with too many extras, because it will cost you in terms of money and possibly in usability.

Only you can weigh the cost/benefit ratio and make a decision.

As you're agonizing over the decision, please realize that "one pack does not a hiker make".

You'll want to have a wardrobe of packs if the hiking bug bites hard. I don't even want to tell you how many packs I have, or how many I've worn out! (You'd need all of your fingers and some of your toes to keep track.)

Channel my little voice in your ear, saying "If it feels right, buy it."

Check in with yourself by putting the pack on one more time, look in the mirror, and...

remember the take home message:

Whichever pack you purchase will have its flaws.

There are always flaws!

So don't procrastinate buying a pack, and don't get angry at yourself if your purchase isn't 100% perfect.

It's all part of learning about hiking gear.

And if you checked into the return & exchange policy, you might have some wiggle room for improvement.

If you're really hesitant to purchase a pack at this time, why not rent one?

Or borrow one?

It's the best way to get to know the features and benefits of each brand.

And you won't feel bad about getting a little mud on the tires, so to speak. Someone ahead of you already did that!

NOW WHAT?

Check in time: How do you feel about buying a pack now?

If you still have a quick question, you can email me.

Another option is to spend 15, 30, 45 or 60 minutes with me on the phone.

If you are vacillating between 2 packs, maybe all you need is to talk it through with me. I can play the devil's advocate almost as well as I play the accordion (no joke! I really do enjoy pounding out a good polka).

Email me to set up a "gear consult" phone call.

If you live in the greater Seattle area, we can meet at your favorite (or soon to become favorite) gear store and I'll not only talk you through your choices, but be sure the pack fits you and fits your needs. A quick email will get this process started.

How much fun would it be to go gear shopping! Yeehaw! Almost as good as hiking, right?

Bonus Chapter Summed Up

Be honest about what kind of hiking you're going to do.

Size up how much gear (i.e weight and volume) you will put in your pack.

Whittle all of the possibilities down to a list of "must have" features.

Comparison shop on line before going to a gear store.

Create a list and/or spreadsheet of "must have" features.

Shop with that data in hand.

Try on packs until you're convinced of a good fit at a good price.

Bring a buddy to help make pack adjustments, or rely upon the availability of a knowledgeable salesperson.

Adopt a "no regrets" attitude toward your purchase. Every pack will teach you something about hiking, and if it really doesn't work out, return it and start over on your quest.

THE END

I really mean it this time.

It's been a pleasure pulling together all of the best hiking tips for you.

Please reach out to me with your comments, suggestions, questions, hiking photos, inspiring quotes, and any other nice thing you'd like to send my way! The HFH website has multiple ways to reach me, including a Contact link in the navigation bar plus an Ask A Question link.

And if you can find the time to write an Amazon review of this book, you would make me one very happy hiker!

My wish for you is **Happy Trails Always**. And **All Ways**.

Diane Spicer

Don't forget, Hiking For Her has social media pages at Facebook, Pinterest and Instagram. Stop by and say hi!

Made in the USA
Coppell, TX
03 December 2021